EMPOWER YOUR NURSING LEADERSHIP

*A Comprehensive Guide to Career Advancement
and Positive Work Environments*

Brandy Covington

Contents

Introduction

In the landscape of every hospital where the hurried footsteps and the subtle sound of machines rule in the spacious hallways, there breathes and strives a quiet force that not only sustains but also participates in the well-being and health care of others. This quiet force is none other than your nursing leadership. Imagine a seasoned nurse whose duties confine her to bedside care; however, she discovers a key that unlocks the immense power hidden within herself, allowing her to expand the wings of her influence from patients' rooms to the fabric of her healthcare system. This transformative experience is a testament to the hidden potential within every nurse. It is the very reason that compels us to enter the realm of **"Empower Your Nursing Leadership: A Comprehensive Guide to Career Advancement and Positive Work Environments."**

The pivotal role of nursing leadership is a dynamic force that stems from the core of every nurse's heart and informs the culture of healthcare institutions. It is not something that is reserved for a few selected persons; instead, its seed is present in every nurse. Moreover, It only takes a moment of realization to allow its branches to grow, ultimately benefiting you and your surroundings. Its innate presence can be better comprehended via an example. We all know that the landscape of healthcare is ever-evolving, and thriving in such an environment requires constant and fast adaptability. With the changing machinery and shift timings, you always maintain your agility and efficiency. This attribute of adaptability is the core of your innate leadership skills. In the upcoming chapters, we will begin our journey to unveil the layering to understand the true meaning of nursing leadership, its impact and significance, the set of challenges, and its metamorphic potential.

In the rich and intricate tapestry of nursing leadership, you will find a myriad of transformative benefits waiting to welcome you. Besides being a roadmap to career advancement, this book is your friend, guiding you to embrace personal and professional growth so that you may bring positive change within your working environment. The author of the book, Brandy Covington, believes that leadership starts with the self. Therefore, the first ripple of transformation that you will embrace during this journey will be the confidence to achieve personal as well as professional growth. Through the glimpses into the lives of nurses and leaders, you will be able to find the areas of improvement within yourself. Moreover, the words will help you explore the actual and exceptional leadership qualities within yourself that you were unaware of. The insightful exercises and strategies to navigate the hurdles with your team will prepare you for personal and professional advancement.

Empower Your Nursing Leadership guides you in fostering caring strategies with your patients and equips you with essential supplies. You will learn to advance in your career by formulating a purpose and a set of strategies. For instance, if you are caught in a situation where you have to make a swift decision, you can do so by stepping into the shoes of an influential advocate not only for your colleagues but also for your patients. By applying this strategy, you will climb the stairs of success. With the power of intention and purpose, you will pave your path towards success.

In the intricate tapestry of life, the journey to self-discovery often unfolds in unexpected ways. Let us have a glimpse at the life of the book's author, Brandy Covington; that journey commenced with a dream of becoming a nurse. However, life had other plans, and the reality of the medical world revealed itself in a way that redirected her path. While her initial aspirations of donning a nurse's cap might have shifted, the essence of caring and serving persisted, steering her towards a different avenue within the healthcare realm. Life's unexpected twists led her to a unique vantage point—a role as the owner of a mobile notary service business that serves her community in a multitude of ways, particularly in the realm of real estate transactions. The daily interactions with individuals navigating the intricacies of property transactions have provided her with insights into the diverse facets of people's lives and the importance of clear communication and empathy in any profession.

Belonging to a family of nurses and friends, she has also lived a life as a nurse assistant. Watching and living the realm of healthcare centers closely, she saw the dire need to empower nurses, especially helping them to get in touch with their leadership skills. That is how Covington decided to write this book. Covington is a born leader and has been flying with colors in her personal and professional life. Implementing the treasure of leadership skills, she excels in every aspect of her life. Be it the work of refinancing home loans, the weight and responsibilities that come with the position of being a mother, managing a good business, or having a flair for words and wisdom, she has managed to flourish in every domain. Being a single mother, she opines that every hurdle that comes in the race of life can make you stronger and more successful if you can see it in your mind's eye. As a feminist, she believes that a woman is nothing less than a queen born to reign in her own world. According to her, leadership is found in every person; however, recognizing it becomes paramount. Therefore, she thought of helping women and men embrace these skills through the art of words.

As a single mom, every decision she makes reverberates not only within the confines of her own life but also shapes the world her children will inherit. The responsibilities of parenthood, coupled with the entrepreneurial challenges of juggling contractors and running a mobile notary service business, have further deepened her understanding of leadership, resilience, and the delicate balance required to navigate the complexities of personal and professional life.

Beyond the realms of business and motherhood, Brandy is a content creator during the stolen moments of free time that life graciously grants her. Whether sharing snippets of daily life, insights into entrepreneurship, reflections on the nuances of modern parenting, or just being silly and comical, content creation has become a channel for self-expression and a connection with a wider community.

Now, you might wonder, why a comprehensive guide on nursing leadership from someone who did not follow the traditional nursing trajectory? The answer lies in the belief that leadership is not confined to a specific role or profession—it is a mindset, a set of skills, and a commitment to continuous growth. Brandy's unique journey, encompassing healthcare aspirations, business ownership, single parenthood, and content creation, has woven a tapestry of experiences that contribute to a holistic understanding of leadership.

Before delving into the art of leadership, Covington wants you to remember that nursing leadership is not a luxury but a necessity. It is an essential ingredient that ensures positive career growth, fosters patient care, and propels you to influence your healthcare institution positively. Knitted in the fabric of personal experience and interest, words come to life to inspire millions of people.

Throughout the book, her voice will uplift you to advance in your career. When it comes to leadership, Covington believes that the root of leadership lies in the heart of confidence and resilience. Passing through the hallways of difficulties and adversities, these attributes can help you end the day on a good note. Likewise, through her personal experiences, she believes in adding positive affirmations in your daily life, for it does the trick and leads you towards positive growth. Her aura of positive growth does not limit itself within the boundaries of individual growth; instead, it impacts the surroundings and blooms the work environment as well. She invites you on this journey of empowerment to help you achieve personal and professional growth by visiting the halls adorned by the lights of knowledge and guarded by the hope and confidence to embrace your leadership qualities.

Chapter 1

The Essence of Nursing Leadership

In the changing world of healthcare, leadership in a nursing career is no less than a compass that guides the team during times of sudden challenges. Transcending the chain of orders and instructions, the leadership is a lighthouse that illuminates the road to compassionate bedside care and progressive development of the entire nursing team. Nursing leadership strives not only for success but also for the safety of the healthcare team. This leadership comes into existence when different attributes come together, and the fashioned nursing leadership can vary in style as well.

In this chapter, we will visit the field of nursing leadership that aspires to excellence as well as growth on individual and collective levels.

Exploring Leadership Styles in Nursing:

A leadership style encompasses a leader's traits, attributes, behavior, and strategies when motivating, directing, and managing a team. Different aspects such as values, expertise, experiences, personality traits, and skills shape a leader's style. A suitable leadership style has a significant impact on the efficiency of the leader. Now, you might be wondering about different styles of nursing leadership so that you may find your style. Let us dive into the world of the versatility of leadership styles.

Nursing leadership entails a variety of styles, each tailored according to the needs of the different healthcare institutions.

Autocratic Leadership:

The autocratic captain of nursing may take the lead during emergency situations to ensure swift decisions in these crucial circumstances.

The autocratic leader does not take any input or advice from the leader; instead, she/he makes all decisions all alone. This type of leadership comes in very handy when implementing zero-occurrence policies.

Democratic Leadership:

Likewise, a democratic navigator implements the collaborative approach to problem-solving by inculcating the input of the whole team.

For example, as a nurse leader, you like to get your team's feedback before making a decision.

Transformation Leadership:

Transformation leaders or true visionaries who motivate their teams to surpass the barriers, chase excellence, and hence achieve collective excellence.

Situational Leadership:

This type of leadership believes in analyzing a situation, until a good approach is unveiled to cultivate the desired positive results. Moreover, this style has some aspects of other leadership styles and is quite adaptable.

For instance, according to the requirements of the situation, a situational leader sometimes becomes very directive. At the same time, that very same leader turns into a supportive one if the situation demands.

Laissez-faire Leadership:

Derived from the French language, it means, allow to do (Saddler, 2023). New and inexperienced nurse leaders prefer this style as it helps them avoid mistakes and errors in their work. This approach is also known as the hands-off approach, and the managers provide neither enough direction nor feedback to their teams, allowing them to function without enough supervision.

As this leadership focuses on individual and independent work, it may be best suited for those who are highly experienced and knowledgeable in their field.

Transactional Leadership:

This leadership style is characterized by focusing on tasks, rewards, and punishments. The leader believes in empowering the team members by gifting them rewards if they perform well and follow every protocol.

This leadership style is best for maintaining protocols and embracing certain tasks; however, it may not help much in inculcating creativity in the team members.

Servant Leadership:

As the name indicates, servant leaders believe in serving and supporting their crew and prioritizing their needs and demands. Servant leadership is marked by empathy, collaboration, compassion, and collective dedication to professional development, and the well-being of each other.

In the field of nursing, this leadership style can help in forming a supportive and creative work ecosystem, filled with the aura of trust and teamwork.

Each of the above-stated styles is a unique approach that allows nursing leaders to lead effectively through the intricate winds of patient care. After choosing your leadership style, you can change the course of your action as well. This begs the question: How to find a leadership style that will suit you?

You can always explore your leadership style in three steps. First, you need to have a clear vision of your goals and tasks. It is through the art of clear goals that you can communicate your vision effectively with your team. To communicate with your team, you need to align that envisioned goal with a particular leadership style and bring it to life through the power of experimentation. You will find your suitable style only through experimentation. For example, you can wear the cloak of transactional leadership to deal with a situation, and if you see that it aligns with your goal and your nature, it is your leadership style.

Before adopting any style, know that leadership is not about perfection at all. Instead, leadership is about leading people with authenticity and honesty.

To know your style, you will also have to cross the land protected by a lot of hurdles. However, by using the right tactics and skills, you will be able to pass through these hurdles easily. A nurse leader has a treasure trove of competencies that are essential to drive their career toward success. You can implement different approaches in your professional life to fly with colors. For example, effective and open communication enables you to design a clear road map that not only helps the crew members understand their roles but also ensures success. On the other hand, as a leader, emotional intelligence will help you to understand and connect with the team's feelings and issues. These feelings will help you to make sound decisions that are beneficial to everyone, hence leading to collective success. Likewise, adaptability is the key to maintaining a seamless course of success. All these qualities work better and more effectively when you, as a leader, show a long-term commitment and dedication towards your team and its goals.

In the bustling corridors of St. Mercy Hospital, a nurse tackled the changing weather of the hospital with a transformative touch. Nurse Leader Tirsa recognized the need for innovative patient care and wore the uniform of a transformational leader. She shared her vision with her team and fueled her team to attain that excellence through communication. One of the challenges that she had to overcome was the restructuring of the hospital's triage system. The leader, Tirsa, knew that the shift would require procedural and cultural change. Therefore, she shared her idea with her team and enlightened them about the benefits of the change and its impact on their workflow. She also acknowledged the doubts and fears of her team members and addressed those doubts and fears with empathy, logical reasoning, and understanding.

During this period of evolution, Tirsa was nothing less than a great leader who became the face of resilience and adaptability when the calamity of resistance prevailed. She also managed to foster a healthy work environment by guiding her team to focus on continuous learning and improving themselves.

The outcomes were extraordinary. The patient care and satisfaction scores multiplied and the reputation of the hospital changed for the good. The efforts of the great leader not only changed the triage system but also positively impacted the culture of the entire nursing unit.

This one example talks about the challenge of embracing change; however, in the realm of nursing managers, you will have to face many challenges.

In essence, knowing your leadership style, embracing its key competencies, and implementing these strategies in real life can help you make a difference in your professional life successfully. Let us delve further to find out how various nurse leaders made an impact in the vast field of nursing.

Case Studies of Successful Nursing Leaders:

Meet Sarah Blake, an experienced nurse with the cloak of compassion and empathy who found herself trapped under the weight of heavy responsibilities. One day, while passing through the intricate maze of patient care, a sudden realization embraced her. At that very moment, she knew that she had the potential to surpass the landscape of computer machines into the spacious halls of healthcare. Sarah's journey mirrors the very metamorphosis that innumerable nurses experience when they unlock the potential hidden in the core of their being - to become a leader. Through the art of her leadership skills, Sarah not only advocated for healthy changes but also inspired her colleagues to do the same. Her leadership helped her design the best positive and productive work environment. This career progress entails the journey of her personal and professional transformation.

Besides this, the art of leadership does not believe in confining itself to the crowns of titles or hierarchical positions. The example of Ruth Lubic is inspiring and moving. Through the armor of nursing leadership, Lubic informed healthcare institutions by fashioning the first free-standing birth center in New York in 1975. Later, in

2002, the Family Health and Birth Center was founded in Washington, DC as well (Wood, 2021).

No discussion about leadership in the realm of nursing is complete without mentioning the Mother of Nursing, Florence Nightingale. She is one of the pioneers who opened the door for modern nursing leadership. During the Crimean War, Nightingale changed the chaotic, unsanitary, and dirty military hospitals into clean and efficient hospitals. Surpassing the conventional mode of nursing, she managed to form the foundation for evidence-based nursing practices through her dedication.

According to Florence, her success story owes to her dedication: "I attribute my success to this – I never gave or took any excuse(Florence)."

Her leadership involved a long-term commitment to patient care and dedication to achieving improved healthcare institutions. Her legacy gifts hope and inspiration to the nurses present all around the globe and asks them to focus on the significance of compassion, empathy, resilience, advocacy, and strategic thinking in the vast and intricate land of leadership.

The book of Past and the Present is filled with many female figures who serve as a beacon of light for all those nurses who are trying to attain successful leadership skills. One such contemporary seminal figure is Dame Betty Kershaw. Throughout her career, she has shown dedication to the importance of advanced nursing education and career development. Skilled in psychiatric nursing, Kershaw explored the importance of advanced degrees, continuous education, and the cloak of adaptation in the demanding healthcare environment.

She not only advocated for higher and advanced standards of education for nurses but also shared her role in the elevation of nursing as a respected and fine profession. Her role as the president of the Royal College of Nursing allowed her to shape policies that helped nurses gain recognition and respect in healthcare institutions.

Another accomplished and well-renowned nurse leader is Dr. Beverly Malone, who has impacted and influenced the art of nursing leadership globally. Her career entails her advocacy for diversity and her leadership positions in several healthcare institutions, including but not limited to being the CEO of the National League for Nursing and the Royal College of Nursing in the United Kingdom.

Malone's leadership, just like Nightingale's, is pregnant with her dedication and commitment to diversity and inclusivity, acknowledging a representative workforce's significance in forming advanced healthcare systems. Trespassing the roadblocks of challenges, she talked about systematic challenges and advised her community to embrace diversity as a prize through her advocacy work. She believes: "Everybody's human, and when it comes to nurses, we can work with everybody (Malone)."

Mary Eliza Mahoney earned the title of the first African-American licensed nurse and became one of the first graduates of the nursing program in 1879 from the New England Hospital for Women and Children. Her journey toward successful leadership is characterized by the armor of resilience, commitment, and determination.

Her commitment to equal rights for people of every race surpasses her personal accomplishments. In 1908, Mahoney co-founded the National Association of Colored Graduate Nurses (NACGN) as well. Her efforts have successfully demolished the walls of barriers and opened the gate to include diversity in the vast land of nursing leadership. Her efforts serve as a guidebook for the present and the future generation of nurses to strive for excellence and success by overlooking their backgrounds.

A distinguished nurse leader not only contributed to nursing education and policies but also brought innovations in nursing curriculum and the field of research; Dr. Claire M. Fagin also became the first female dean of the University of Pennsylvania School of Nursing, where she informed a lot of healthcare policies. Likewise, the height of her leadership career extended to national levels, where she served on committees and advisory boards to help bring positive change to healthcare policies.

As she advocated for pursuing advanced nursing degrees, she also addressed the need to practice advanced nursing roles to strive in the competitive field of healthcare. Her efforts encompassing the correspondence of academia, research, and policy adherence speak for the systemic change that nurse leaders can bring to any healthcare institution. Her leadership style is a perfect example of systemic change.

One of the fine examples demonstrating the significance of nurses' roles in challenging times compels us to meet Dr. Margaret Chan. From 2007 to 2017, She served as the Director-General of the World Health Organization (WHO). Her leadership skills, comprising effective communication, collaboration, and strategic approach, have become the leading example of democratic leadership. She dealt with all the challenges of global health crises, such as H1N1 influenza and the outbreak of the Ebola virus, effectively and strategically.

In the shadow of her leadership, WHO worked on the health system strengthening, preparing them to face the upcoming pandemics and addressing health-related concerns. Like many other nurse leaders, she recognized the importance of nursing education and encouraged the nurses to invest in their education so that they may contribute to public health initiatives.

The journey of these nursing leaders, from past figures like Florence Nightingale to contemporary ones such as Dame Betty Kershaw, shows a variety of pathways that a nurse can take to make a long-lasting impact and contribute to the well-being and success of nursing landscapes. All of these tales become the beacon of inspiration for those nurses who want to contribute to the world of health care and a guidebook for those leaders who need direction and guidance to climb the mountains of hurdles smoothly. In essence, by providing tangible insights, along with strategic career planning, the stories live to help nurses strive for excellence.

Practical Leadership Tips:

Effective healthcare leadership requires a set of expertise and attributes to deal with the intricacies of healthcare environments successfully. Having said that, let us explore some of the practical tips and tactics that you can inculcate in your professional lives to multiply the effectiveness in target regions, such as communication and personal and professional growth.

The Cornerstone of Leadership:

The cornerstone of leadership is effective communication. Timely communication with active listening can help you overcome obstacles prevailing on the road to professional success. An effective communication tool also brings unity among the team members.

Maintain a Balance Between Speed and Precision:

As nurse leaders, you will have to make swift and accurate decisions under a lot of pressure. You can make sound decisions by evaluating the risks, outcomes, and advantages of every possible decision. It is always wise to look ahead and evaluate the consequences if the circumstances may vary in the future.

You can also make a good decision by involving your team's perspective. Let their valuable insights influence your thoughts and decision-making skills efficiently. Likewise, a sound decision births from the root of sound knowledge. Therefore, a good nurse leader keeps on learning and believes in staying up-to-date with the latest trends in the industry.

All these tools will help you make sound decisions on time.

Team Collaboration:

Through team collaboration, a nurse leader, along with her team can touch the heights of the sky. You can foster a productive environment by valuing each member of your team and encouraging their efforts and accomplishments. You can enhance the rate of success of your unit by providing effective and constructive feedback to each member of your team.

Adaptability:

The cloak of adaptability will help you conquer the world in every aspect of your life. In the field of nursing, to join hands with adaptability, you will have to embrace change quickly, see challenges as opportunities for growth, and cultivate resilience.

Self-Care:

The importance of self-care in any phase of life is as important as the life itself. Dedication, commitment, and effort become useless if you do not take care of yourself. A nurse leader must prioritize her health and well-being over everything if she wants to achieve and maintain success.

As the road to success is both challenging and time-consuming, you will need good health to pass these hurdles. You can manage your health by setting boundaries and forming a balance between your work and personal life. Please take the necessary rest and avoid the long-lasting exhaustion resulting from working constantly. Do not confuse commitment and dedication with working without a break and rest. Likewise, invest your spare time in those activities that help you rejuvenate your health and mind. For example, you can spend your time with your friends, relatives, and friends to restore mental freshness.

Successful nursing leadership is a process of continuous efforts and struggles. It starts at the moment when you make up your mind to work on yourself. If you need any tips or strategies to help you reach the success of your dreams, you can implement the above-mentioned practical tips that are best suited for your journey. But, let the seed of self-care grow in every nurse's toolkit.

Time To Take The Test:

Before we continue our journey, stop here and take a self-assessment test to get to know your existing leadership skills, your strengths, and areas of improvement. This evaluation will be the first initiative toward your effective leadership development odyssey.

- ↔ You can draw two columns (either on paper or on a digital notepad) titled 'Strengths' and 'Weaknesses.'

- ↔ Now, write all your strong points, such as effective communication, under the category 'Strengths.' Likewise, write all of your weak points, like lack of confidence, under the category 'Weaknesses.'

- ↔ All the points under the category of Weaknesses are the areas of your improvement.

As you have explored several leadership styles and have visited the lives of impactful nurse leaders, you can not only identify your leadership style but also envision your future in leadership.

In the upcoming chapter, we will delve deep into the land of strategies necessary to overcome all the challenges and issues that may stand before us on this journey toward success.

Let's resume our journey toward success and empowerment in the spacious and challenging world of nursing leadership by unlocking our leaders within ourselves.

Chapter 2

Navigating Career Challenges in Nursing

No journey to success is without its challenges and obstacles. The same is the case with nursing leadership. The journey to effective and successful nursing leadership passes from the stations of hurdles and obstacles that seem paramount to cross. However, these hurdles are nothing but a stepping stone towards the destination of your success. If you are looking for ways to turn your workplace obstacles and struggles into success, dive into the world of words that will help you navigate your challenges, and a Master of Science in Nursing (MSN) degree will let you see the challenges as mere opportunities for growth and development.

Identifying Career Growth Opportunities:

In the spacious realm of nursing, the career opportunities are as diverse as the patients you care for. While passing through the hallways of your hospital, you know that the height of your success is not bounded by the walls of a hospital; instead, it extends to the realms of various advanced degrees, diplomas, and certifications. Besides that, it involves the touch of specialized training, along with your vision of a successful future.

Just like varying leadership styles, growth opportunities have different types. According to your taste and innate skills, you can identify where your chance lies. By identifying your growth opportunities, you will be able to climb the stairs of success strategically.

Like any other profession, the growth in the nursing profession starts from education. By selecting a particular degree or course, you can design a smooth roadmap toward success founded on your interests and tastes.

If your heart yearns for the nursing leader position, you can pursue a Master of Science in Nursing (MSN) degree. The degree will take you into the world of knowledge and Science. With the help of a degree, you can open the door to many different roles, including but not limited to a practitioner specializing in family, acute care, or pediatric care. In addition to that, it helps you unlock the door of nursing leadership.

The anchor of Doctor of Nursing Practice (DNP) helps in solidifying your expertise. You can not only embrace expertise in polishing your clinical skills but also transform yourself into a trailblazer - impacting and informing the research, healthcare policies, and their implementation. This degree prepares you to become a skilled leader in the vast career of nursing.

When discussing the opportunities leading to the success of leadership, certificates are the flags that can be hoisted with pride and confidence. Critical Care Registered Nurse (CCRN) propels you as a nurse to leave your leadership mark in times of critical and sensitive scenarios. For example, it is through the art of this certificate that you prove yourself worthy of handling the intricacy of high-acuity patient scenarios.

Certified Clinical Research Professional (CCRP) warmly welcomes you with open hands if your inclination is toward the rhythmic melody of a beating heart. Through the cloak of cardiovascular nursing, you not only show care for your patients but also tailor cardiac rehabilitation programs to enlighten a path of recovery and well-being for your patients.

If you plan to achieve an executive position, Nurse Executive Advanced Certification (NEA-BC) certification will help you achieve your goal. The course is fashioned by keeping in mind the role of leadership; therefore, it equips you with leadership tools, including but not limited to management, strategic planning, and resilience to navigate through the challenging times of healthcare institutions.

It is through these certificates and degrees that you assert your specialty, expertise, and credibility in the vast hallways of the healthcare ecosystem. Suffice it to say that both of them are the first step that leads you to embrace long-lasting success.

Near the realm of degrees and certificates lies an entity that focuses on the practical implementation of leadership and management skills. This entity is none other than training programs. These programs help you to advance seamlessly through the dubious and threatening currents of the healthcare system. Advanced training programs, such as Advanced Cardiovascular Life Support (ACLS) and Pediatric Advanced Life Support (PALS), provide the tools of critical thinking and confidence to future nurse leaders so that they may face all kinds of hardships with a smile on their faces.

Engrained in the universal and global perspectives, the International Board Certified Lactation Consultant (IBCLC) is another advanced training program that emphasizes making an impact through the potential of knowledge and guidance. Through this training program, you will be able to make a difference in maternal and child health. Your wisdom, combined with your knowledge, will guide others to navigate the challenges of breastfeeding by promoting the infant's well-being and the mother's health.

The beauty of success lies in personalized navigation between the vast landscape of opportunities. You have the power to form your recipe for success. You can amalgamate a Master's in MSN Ed, Certified Nurse Educator (CNE), and specialized training to reach your goals. For instance, you can attain CNE certification, along with pursuing a master's in MSN Ed, and become a beam of hope and transformation for the coming generations of nursing.

As the road to success is non-linear, you can always choose to move forward by assessing and evaluating the scope of your aspirations and goals. In this advancing journey, if you see a spark of another aspiration or goal tingling in your mind, you can research the future of that particular aspiration and align your passion accordingly.

In short, the chances and prospects of growth in nursing are as vast as the diagnosis in the medical field. This impactful journey is more than professional growth and evolution; it is a testament to the unwavering resilience, power of dedication, and force of commitment of nurses who aim to shape the future of nursing as well so that you may keep on flourishing the healthcare ecosystem.

Strategies for Professional Development:

With the evolving landscape of nursing, the heart of professional development lies in constant efforts. The journey requires a plethora of strategies that help in advancing toward professional growth. From the skills of networking to the art of mentorship and the corridors of conferences and workshops, you can adopt actionable strategies so that you may keep on flourishing.

The power of networking in any aspect of life cannot be undermined. It is a focal point that binds the community of nurses together. In this world of professional connections, a support system comes to life that helps all to endure the concerns and obstacles of the healthcare community. Engaging yourself in online as well as offline professional organizations can teach you a lot of things. For example, through these organizations and meetings, you can share your experiences, listen to the insights of your community fellows, and access a pool of collective beneficial knowledge.

You can find these organizations everywhere, especially in the ruling era of the digital world. One such platform is LinkedIn, where a community of nurses showcases their skills, builds a link with other colleagues, drinks the syrup of knowledge regularly, and stays updated on the latest trends in their field. These connections contribute to potential career growth as well. Ultimately, such connections become the source of guidance, advice, and mentorship.

Hence, fashioning a network is more than forming contacts; it is about forming relationships that add to mutual growth.

Along the path of professional development, the mentors keep on guiding their mentees. Be it climbing the early stairs of a nursing career or championing the intricacies rooted in the path to leadership, a mentor can offer you help and guidance. The expert or mentor serves as a useful insight during times of difficulty.

Even in healthcare institutions, you can join formal mentorship programs. Whenever you face any difficulty, you can look at these mentors who have the potential to help you by providing useful pieces of wisdom. However, the aim of mentorship is not confined to you. For example, you, as a mentee, instill the pearls of wisdom received from your mentors into your brain, and in return, you become the vessel of change; you contribute to new perspectives, technological insights, and the collective growth of the entire community. Having said that, both parties advance toward development just through the mutual act of serving.

Let us now meet a nurse who is about to become a Nurse manager. Her upcoming position requires the amalgamation of clinical skills and management expertise. However, she lacks in management skills. Therefore, she decides to get useful pieces of advice and guidance from her mentor. This guidance will help her become the head of her unit and help her team grow through mentorship skills. When she uses these skills, she will be adding her efforts to the whole system, resulting in collective success.

To advance in the professional domain, the significance of attending conferences and workshops needs to be highlighted as well. If you attend these conferences and workshops, you absorb practical wisdom, learn insights, keep an eye on the latest trends, and adopt actionable strategies in one go. You can always benefit from attending national conferences and online international conferences as they invite the best speakers and leaders advancing in the same field.

These conferences and workshops also help you to establish and join a network. Hence, it unites the nurses who are on the same page as you are, making the connections real and successful.

If you examine closely, you will identify that these tools provide you with a chance to invest in yourself. By investing your time in conferences and workshops, you can not only unlock your hidden potential but can touch the sky by polishing your skills.

As the needs of healthcare keep on changing, continuing education can help you attain your goals and aspirations. In this advanced world of digital land, pursuing education in your profession is no longer a barrier. Many universities and health institutions offer advanced degrees, such as MSN or DNP, while allowing nurses to continue their professional commitment. These certifications and degrees promise excellence in your career. You can pursue education through online webinars, classes, and conferences as well.

All the modes of career and professional advancement are about sharing knowledge. One such useful tool for passing on your wisdom and knowledge is publishing papers. Writing articles or publishing research papers can contribute to healthcare publications as they share invaluable insights and strengthen your position as a thoughtful leader. If you find out that writing is not your best ally, no worries; you can participate in publishing research papers by editing or doing the research work. Remember that the goal of research is to polish your skills by learning and using the lens of investigation. These skills of research and experimentation will come in handy in the future as well. Moreover, you can always share your ideas or information via blogs, articles, and social media posts.

As you embark on this journey of professional development, it is essential to understand that this growth is a holistic approach to development rather than being a chain of separate activities. These different forms of learning aim toward one goal, that is, mutual and individual growth. So, start your journey towards long-term success.

But, before that, it is important to acknowledge that you cannot use all of these options. All you need to do is to find out the best form of learning according to your aspirations and passion. In the next step, stick to that strategy and begin to pave your road toward success.

Overcoming Workplace Challenges:

Sometimes, do you feel that your workplace challenges are stopping you from attaining your career dreams? At the same time, you have the urge to fight these challenges. So, use that urge to prepare yourself to overcome career obstacles and experience genuine professional growth. On your way, the cap of leadership will help you achieve your goals quite seamlessly. When it comes to the profession of nursing, it is no lie that nursing is more than a profession. It is a vocation that desires leadership by encompassing the technical skills and knowledge of the medical landscape.

As a nurse leader, you will have to deal with challenges as complex as complex diagnoses in the intricate landscape of health care. The issues and challenges can be damaging communication gaps present in the interdepartmental teams, rightful yet threatening demands of quality care, or the shortage of staff. You can face these challenges by acknowledging them as the first step leading to the destination of healthy growth rather than finding them fearful obstacles.

To cope with these challenges, you can wear the uniform of innovation. Picture yourself as a strategist who uses technology to enhance communication with your colleagues and members. You can ensure that your crew is neither underutilized nor overwhelmed by employing optimization systems for the nurse-patient ratio (similar to precision instruments). Likewise, the thoughtful use of telehealth will provide you with a lifeline for staff and patients alike. Navigating through the intricate web of challenges, the cloak of resilience can always come in handy.

Meet Nurse Amanda, who dealt with the obstacles through her positive attitude. When she came across the issue of short staff, Amanda did not feel terrified of these circumstances; instead, she got up and looked for strategies to tackle this unforeseen situation. She started a mentorship program that granted her team not only the embryo of confidence but also the spirit to fight this situation together. Her story is a reflection of the transformative power of mentorship in a nursing career.

Another life story of the leader nurse, Bongi Sibanda, is not only filled with struggles but also with the dedication to achieve her goals. Her story is an inspiration for us all. According to Sibanda, her secret to success is her dedication and resilience (Hannah Nightingale 2020, 2019). When she started working in the vast realm of nursing, she had to work twice as hard compared to her colleagues. Not only that, she had to prove herself in the field of advanced clinical practice. Coming from a BME (Black and Minority Ethnic) background, it took her a lot of hard work to prove her worth. However, no obstacle was big enough in front of her mighty spirit and resilience.

By looking at the glimpses of these figures, It would not be wrong to say that the challenges and issues handled by the nurse leaders are nothing but mere opportunities to grow in the healthcare department. It is through these innovative approaches that you can transform the obstacles into opportunities.

Whenever you find yourself entangled in the web of challenges, take a deep breath and try to design a roadmap of causes and consequences. Through this approach, you can pick the course of action that will generate the best positive outcomes in the long haul. The consequences or the impact of your actions will touch the realm of patient care, surpassing your aura.

What comes to your mind when you think of a good leader? I am sure that the answer will involve establishing positive relationships and building lasting collaborations. By visiting the hallways of practical wisdom and strategies, you will be able to open the wide door leading to the success of your institution as well as your career. The words of empathy and kindness will lead you to form healthy and positive relationships with your team, colleagues, and interdisciplinary teams so that you may become a true and successful leader.

As you start to inculcate positive energy and efforts into your work, a positive outcome in the form of success or growth starts to originate. This positive outcome grants you more energy and satisfaction. Surpassing the realm of your professional life, a positive attitude and satisfaction enter your personal life, too. You can enhance this tint of satisfaction and happiness by aligning your personal life with your professional values and leadership approach. The practice of self-reflection welcomes you to get an understanding of your goals, motivations, and aspirations. By learning the art of self-reflection (what do you want), you will be able to conquer your personal as well as professional lives.

It is a well-known belief that a positive and healthy workspace is a myth. In reality, the work environment mirrors difficulties, toxicity, and stagnancy. But what if the concept of a positive work environment can become a reality? Through inculcating the best patient care and professional growth in your hospital setting, you can fashion and foster a long-lasting positive health environment. As a nurse manager, you can forge a healthy environment thriving on respect, open communication, and teamwork. You can also establish a healthy workspace by employing these tools. Also, through the implementation of these strategies, not only will you fly high with colors, but your entire team will too.

Mastering the art of advocacy is one of the powerful approaches to nursing leadership. Be it championing your teams' rights, winning the right demands of your patients, or implementing the policy changes in your nursing realm; you can use the art of voice or advocacy to bring constructive and productive transformation. Along with benefitting your team, your voice will benefit the larger systems within the sphere of healthcare.

Resilience is one of the best cloaks that one can wear while navigating through the challenges of life. Likewise, the quality of resilience is no less than a powerful antidote when it comes to facing the hurdles in your professional growth. Each phase of your career encompasses a set of challenges, and the phase of leadership is also one of them. It poses continuous hurdles and challenges in your path toward success. The hurdles empower you to battle these challenges through the art of resilience. It helps you to fight the germs of these obstacles by showing the power of resilience and by providing you an insight into the obstacles with their solutions. The skill of resilience will also help you establish a productive work-life balance.

We will talk about resilience in detail in the coming chapters as well.

Time To Set Your Goals:

Let us learn to apply the above practices to our practical lives.

- ↔ One fun and useful way to design your roadmap to success is via a goal-setting exercise.

- ↔ In this exercise, your pieces of equipment will be your mind, a piece of paper or a digital notepad, and a pen.

- ↔ First, take a deep breath and start thinking about all your goals. After thinking, you need to write these goals onto your paper.

- ↔ Next, turn the page and draw two long boxes. One will be reserved for short-term goals; while the other for long-term goals.

➻ In the last step, by revising your goals written on the last page, you will identify the short-term and long-term goals and put them in their respective boxes.

Hint: Short-term goals are those goals that can be achieved in a short span of time. For example, learning the art of effective communication. However, long-term goals refer to those long-lasting goals that require a lot of time and effort. For instance, becoming a nurse leader is a long-term goal.

This very exercise has become your map for your professional development.

Knowing the ways to overcome your work-life obstacles and strengthening your skills, you are well-equipped to move forward. In the next chapter, we will explore and discuss the specifics of overcoming workplace challenges.

As you continue your journey through the pages, the practical strategies will welcome you, and you will see that the aspiration that seems distant has always been within your reach. So, let us continue empowering ourselves.

Chapter 3

Overcoming Workplace
Challenges for Nursing Leaders

Imagine a work ecosystem where the obstacles, concerns, and intricacies are not considered roadblocks; instead, they are embraced as opportunities for growth and professional development. In the landscape of nursing leadership, battling these challenges and obstacles is paramount. Nursing leaders play a crucial role in ensuring the best quality of patient care most of the time. They have to face the complexities of the team dynamics, analyze these challenges, and implement useful strategies to overcome these challenges. These examples will also help us to adopt these strategies into our lives.

Let us delve into some more useful and realistic strategies to navigate the challenges of the healthcare environment in this very chapter.

Navigating Team Dynamics:

In a healthcare setting, team dynamics entail the art of interactions, the strong bondage of relationships, and the exchange of communication among health professionals. It is impossible to achieve optimal patient care without teamwork in the stressful and advanced healthcare ecosystem. The nursing leaders should try to foster a high-performing and dedicated team by overcoming these challenges.

As a nurse leader, you can motivate your team toward success through the art of communication and the power of actions. The role of effective communication needs to be underscored here, as miscommunication can give birth to misunderstandings, errors, and average patient care. To ensure the collective effort, it becomes mandatory for you to address differences and misunderstandings in communication so that transparency may run in the halls of your organization. You can encourage open dialogue to help your team grow collectively.

To maintain a positive and healthy work ecosystem, it is necessary to discuss and solve some issues and conflicts immediately and, in some cases, in front of everyone. This also serves as a beacon of success and inspiration for others. In addition to that, everyone sees that the team is run by a manager who values equality.

Likewise, collaboration and interdependency are crucial to delivering sublime and best patient-centered care in different healthcare organizations. The leaders must encourage the facilitation of teamwork among physicians, therapists, doctors, and nurses to follow a holistic approach.

Another way to establish networks, collaboration, and interpersonal relationships is to organize team-building activities outside the walls of your healthcare institution.

For example, what will you do if you are unable to find common foundations to form a collaborative ground in your unit?

You can organize regular interdisciplinary meetings or workshops and invite professionals from different branches of various disciplines to join these meetings. In the meetings, you can politely encourage all the professionals to not only share their insights but also discuss multiple patient cases. This initiative will help you to enhance collaboration, along with the success of your whole organization.

Be it any domain of life, the significance of empathy is monumental. An empathetic leader is the backbone of any successful leadership movement. In any healthcare system, especially in the emotional healthcare work system, an empathetic leader is no less than a healing touch. Through empathy, you, as a nursing leader, can listen to your crew actively, gain knowledge of their dilemmas, and grant support when needed.

Imagine this: The clouds of challenging times are spreading over your unit, and your team is having an emotional toll that is affecting their performance. What would you do as a nurse supervisor?

You can always conduct individual meetings to ensure the mental stability of your team members. Also, you can talk to them regarding the situation until they wear the mask of calmness. This approach will also foster a healthy support system within your team.

One of the best strategies to multiply the scores of excellence, fortify the fortress of positive healthcare, and polish the skills is an investment in the professional growth of your team members. Nursing leaders need to identify opportunities that help in the professional development of the individuals as well as the team.

Let us imagine a workspace where your manager has launched a program to acknowledge the contributions of the best performers publicly. When your performance is extraordinary, you receive the gifts of appreciation and accolades publicly. This act of appreciation has boosted your morale and motivated you to work more efficiently. As a result, you start to work more efficiently, which will benefit the entire organization.

Let us implement this therapy of acknowledgment and appreciation into our professional lives. As a nurse leader, you can recognize and celebrate the success of your staff on individual as well as collective levels. It will significantly enhance the morale of your team members.

By applying the strategies of open communication, empathetic approach, professional development, appreciation, and team-building activities, nursing leaders can share their part in painting an environment full of positivity, cohesion, and success.

Effective Communication in Leadership:

In the dubious currents of times, the tool of effective communication becomes no less than a rescuer. It is the power of words that can boost the morale of a person and motivate them to soar in their career.

According to Garcia (2012), "If you can't communicate effectively, you will not lead."

In a professional setting, communication is more than passing information. Instead, communication is a two-way street where you not only speak but also listen to the perspective of your teammates. This two-way street cleans the clutter of unnecessary information and forms a clean and transparent pathway leading to a successful career.

You can enhance your communication skills in the realm of your leadership by joining a training program or by adopting some of these best strategies:

Active Listening:

A good leader always understands the perspectives of her team members through the aid of active listening. The holistic practitioner Laurie Buchanan believes that "When we invest in active listening, the dividend is an expanded capacity for compassion." The tool kit of active listening consists of giving full attention to the concerned members, asking questions if they have some kinds of doubts, and providing constructive and healthy feedback.

Meet Tina, a Nursing manager who always listens to her employees' concerns and encourages feedback during her meetings. She not only listens to the concerns of her team members but also shows the organization's commitment to valuing each and every voice equally.

Transparency:

Transparent communication makes sure that the message is conveyed correctly. It consists of clear and concise communication and the elimination of all the points that can blur the vision of the intended message.

Transparent communication also allows the staff to understand the series of reasoning and thinking behind a particular decision.

Open Communication:

The door to open communication plays a vital role in fostering trust and building interpersonal relationships. A nurse leader must be ready to face success and challenges through the portal of communication. In addition to that, open communication eliminates the differences that can be harmful to an organization.

For example, you, as a nurse leader, communicate with your team members to unveil the reason behind your sudden approach to shift timings in the work environment. Through this open communication, your team members will feel that they are part of the entire organization rather than being only employees. As a result of this realization, you will see them aligning their dedication and goals in a new direction that will cultivate mutual success.

Adaptability in Communication Styles:

When the leaders choose to communicate, you might have noticed that they adopt a particular style of communication. They adjust their tones and adopt a unique style of communication that will mirror their goal of communication.

You can also tailor your communication style based on the individual preferences of your team members. For example, some members respond better to written updates, while others prefer face-to-face interaction. This form of adaptability shows your commitment and value towards your teammates.

The Seed of Empathy in Communication:

A great nurse leader knows the importance of a positive healthcare ecosystem where the patient gets the required dose, as well as empathy. As a nurse leader who believes in collective success, you can always choose to improve your surrounding area by also making the satisfaction of patients active participants in their journey towards health and well-being.

A true leader always wears the mask of empathy as it is one of the most essential tools to advance in both personal and professional life.

When you speak with empathy, you communicate your understanding of your members' emotions, perspectives, and concerns. Thus, the seed of empathy grows in a work realm run by mutual support and efforts.

Take the case of Sabrina, a senior nurse executive who always demonstrates empathy by acknowledging the concerns of her team during a demanding and tiring project. Her communication, full of compassion and empathy, has boosted her team's adaptability, resilience, and morale.

If you can embed this quality into your responsibilities, you will experience a positive and blooming work environment. The kind words of understanding and empathy for one person can brighten up someone's day, which ultimately brings light into your life. Now, imagine that you are considerate of your colleagues, your patients, and their needs. The chances of you making sound and best decisions have multiplied automatically. Your voice of compassion, empathy, and understanding turns into a heartbeat of care that starts to echo in the vast tapestry of your healthcare institution.

The Feedback:

Effective communication regarding a team member's performance involves recognition and appreciation of his strengths and highlighting the areas of improvement in a non-degrading manner. Effective communication believes in delivering the deserved appreciation and constructive feedback to the team members.

The loop of constructive feedback helps a team understand its performance and contribute to its professional growth and development. You can provide feedback to your team to enhance the efficiency rate.

We will discover the healing potential of the feedback in the next chapters as well.

Confidence:

Remember: Confidence is the key.

> "The foundation of self-confidence, the basis of boldness and self-assertion, is a deep inner trust, based on living a life of perfect integrity, and disciplining yourself to live consistent with your highest values in every situation (Tracy, 2012)."

When you, as a leader, speak with confidence, the uttered words become a testament to the truth and surety for the team members. It is through the use of confidence that your members choose to work with you, listen to you, and move toward the road to success.

Effective communication is considered a cornerstone of successful leadership that shapes an organization's culture and cultivates positive outcomes.

In addition to that, your voice gives confidence to others to make a positive change in their work environments by following these kinds of healthy practices. It is the power of your leadership qualities that improves patient outcomes effectively. Most importantly, the journey that you began alone does not end on the same note; instead, many people accompany you along the way, and through collective efforts and innovative approaches, you change the world around you.

Organizational Dynamics and Leadership:

The health industry is quite intricate, and several organizational dynamics immersed within this industry play a critical role in enhancing or worsening the quality of patient care. Besides understanding the complexities of healthcare institutions, effective nursing leadership always requires the potential to inform organizational structures.

From hierarchical dynamics to the orientation of leadership goals with the organizational objectives, let us explore the nuances of organizational dynamics.

To ensure transparent lines of authoritative figures and to ensure that decisions add to the organization's well-being, the healthcare industry chooses hierarchical structures. As the main aim of these structures is to enhance efficiency and effectiveness, sometimes, these structures become hurdles in the pathway of effective communication and teamwork. Successful nursing leaders value the balance between authority and teamwork while maintaining a hierarchical framework.

Time and again, the importance of communication is asserted as it is through language and conversation that we communicate our ideas, goals, and thoughts. Clear and transparent communication helps in conveying correct information throughout the whole organization. Despite being in hierarchical structures, ensure that you encourage your teams to put forth their understanding and feedback so that you may make an informed decision. Involving Frontline staff who directly impact the quality of patient care can be a good idea.

In the leadership dynamics, you will come across some situations where you will have to change your leadership style. If you have knowledge of all the leadership styles, you can win the challenge easily. For instance, during patient care times, if you feel that your democratic leadership style is unable to form a sound impact, you can wear the uniform of authoritative leadership for the time being. In times of crisis, your participative approach has been changed into a directive approach. Hence, this approach is another face of adaptability in the dynamic world of leadership.

We have also learned that successful nursing leadership is interconnected with the need for individual leadership objectives. In other words, the interconnectedness of short-term goals with long-term goals. But why is this alignment significant in the realm of nursing?

This alignment of interconnectedness ensures a collaborative, cohesive, and harmonious approach to embracing the whole organization's mission and its success.

Let us understand this interconnectedness through an exercise.

Imagine that you always find yourself on the frontlines serving the patients as an emphatic and compassionate healer in the bustling halls of nursing. Close your eyes and visualize all the moments that mean success to you- a patient's peaceful smile, a discovery in the field of medical research, or a staff that resonates with the rhythm of collaboration to achieve shared goals.

With the visions in your mind, start to design your pathway toward a successful leader by thinking of your career plan as a map leading you toward your ultimate goal. You can break down your main goal into little achievable landmarks (short-term). These landmarks can be educational progress or personal growth. By passing through these landmarks, you attain your ultimate goal, that is, to become a successful nurse leader.

In simple words, this approach of interconnectedness becomes a strategic imperative.

However, you, as a nurse manager, can lead to the success of the whole organization only if you have a clear understanding of the goals and vision of your healthcare institute. This first body of knowledge helps you form sound decisions that will capture the long-term achievements and visions of your career and organization.

We are discussing the long-term success of your nursing leadership career. However, what do we mean when we use the term 'long-term' success?

Long-term success can be better comprehended through the example of changing weather. Be it the season of harsh cold winds or the excruciating heat; you try to avoid direct contact with them because your health can wither easily. This strategy benefits you in both winter and summer. In the ever-evolving land of nursing, changes keep on knocking on the door. Sometimes, it is the changing policies, and other times; it is the changing types of machinery. To maintain the stability (long-term success) of implementing decisions along with the success of the whole institution, it is mandatory to envision the possibility of changes and upcoming challenges.

While long-term sustainability and success are the goal, short-term goals can be helpful in this race as well. You cannot only check the chances of long-term goals but also implement immediate changes with the help of short-term goals. However, the balance between short-term and long-term can be achieved via foresighting situations.

The heartbeat of any organization is its institutional culture that determines how people interact with each other and work together. You, as a nurse manager, have the potential to impact and shape the workplace's culture, cultivating a friendly aura to promote collaboration, creativity, and enhanced patient care.

You can refine your work environment by adopting certain strategies. You can lead by setting an example. When nursing leaders embody the qualities and principles that they want in their team, they not only create an environment of authenticity and trust but also automatically get the desired results in a shorter period. Similarly, empowering individuals to offer their suggestions and feedback regarding patient care can lead to an environment where continuous improvement thrives. When you are empowering your team by valuing their suggestions, occasions to celebrate come into existence. Celebrating each victory (small and large) can also enhance effectiveness and motivate everyone to work more efficiently. To welcome the air of change in the corridors of your organization, equip your staff members with essential training and resources. This proactive strategy makes sure that the team is ready for all the upcoming challenges, such as changes in healthcare policies and practices.

In the fascinating yet intricate world of nursing and healthcare in general, organizational dynamics and leadership must go hand-in-hand. Through the strategies of effective communication, knowledge, adaptability, active listening, and empathy, you as a nurse manager can not only lead to success of your own but also contribute to influencing the whole organization. By mastering these skills, your team is bound to offer top-notch patient-centered care.

Time to Practice Role-Play Scenarios (An Activity) :

To ensure that you perform well in challenging times as a nurse leader, let us practice through role-play scenarios.

- ↔ Envision all the challenges that may come across in a workplace setting. For instance, you are having problems dealing with machinery.

- ↔ Now, try to raise questions and objections with your manager as a team member.

- ↔ Next, step into the shoes of a nurse leader and try to answer all the questions with the best possible solutions and examples. Try to communicate all the policy changes with your teammates effectively and clearly.

- ↔ During the activity, maintain the pressure of the situation accordingly.

This exercise in a controlled environment will prepare you to employ effective communication skills and leadership tools in real-life scenarios as effectively as possible.

As you learn to conquer the intricacies of workplace issues, you are not merely mastering skills but also making sure that you become a successful nurse leader.

In the next chapter, let us learn about the proactive leadership that will help you foster a great positive work culture.

Chapter 4

Proactive Leadership for Positive Work Environments

Would it not be amazing to not only navigate safely through the land of obstacles but also form a workplace where excellence strives? In this chapter, we will unravel the transformative potential of proactive leadership that will equip you with tools to fashion a healthy and innovative work environment. These proactive strategies will also enable you to shape an empowering work culture.

Forming a positive work culture is in the hands of an aspiring leader, and it is not as difficult as it sounds. As a true nurse leader, you can create an innovative work environment by implementing a set of proactive leadership skills.

But before everything, It is important to familiarize ourselves with the concept of a work culture.

A work culture entails a set of values, beliefs, and behaviors that guide an institution. It forms a peculiar set of expectations for how individuals should behave and interact with each other while fulfilling their day-to-day duties and sharing their roles for the greater benefit of the whole organization.

You can create a positive work culture by:

Developing a Sense of Belonging:

A positive culture stems from a sense of belonging where individuals feel that they are an integral part of the whole association.

As a nurse leader, you can create this feeling in a lot of ways. First of all, you can create a sense of belonging by demonstrating inclusivity through a series of actions and policies. The actions may involve making the whole team feel appreciated and recognized for their distinctive contributions despite belonging to different ethnicities and roles. Similarly, the policies showing the regard for the team members can be useful. Second of all, you, as a nurse leader, can organize team-building seminars, workshops, or activities to fortify professional relationships. In these meetings, you can discuss the current environment as the light on the current environment helps in forming a positive environment. Third of all, you can make your team members realize that they are heard. Last of all, you can make sure that these strategies make the team workers feel respected.

Promoting a Culture that Aims for Excellence:

A positive workplace is built on the foundation of excellence, and therefore, it keeps on striving for excellence. Nurse managers can foster such a culture by providing opportunities to their teams that promise professional growth and development. However, it is not an easy task to offer opportunities without offering insights into these opportunities. The set of insights should encompass proper training, knowledge, or continuous learning. When you are a nurse leader, you need to maintain the distance between your expectations (regarding your team)and your team's work strategies.

You may not need to micromanage every move of your team as it will affect the efficiency of the whole team, and some of the team members can feel insecure too.

The custom of reward and acknowledgment can be a useful proactive leadership strategy as well. Cultivating a rewarding work culture can be comprehended in six steps: Defining brilliance, modeling brilliance, empowering brilliance, challenging brilliance, rewarding brilliance, and maintaining brilliance.

Underscoring Work-Life Balance:

It is no lie that the demanding field of nursing requires a lot of dedication combined with hard work. Visionary leaders always emphasize the well-being of their members through a realistic approach. You can set realistic expectations by communicating them with your team. You can tailor realistic work expectations by considering the physical as well as emotional requirements of your team and the whole nursing profession. You can ask them to avoid burnout due to excessive workloads as it will affect their health and the organization's mission in the long haul.

You can also provide relaxation in their daily routine tasks when possible. It will cheer their mood. As a nurse leader, you will be able to identify the demands of your team and offer chances so that they may balance their personal and professional lives side by side. In the realm of the nursing profession, you can empower the concept of well-being by taking initiatives that address the need for physical and mental health. The initiative can range from stress management resources, and mental health services, to access to health programs.

Strengthening Individual Contributions:

A healthy workplace becomes more positive and innovative when proactive leaders empower and engage with their team members. As an inspirational leader, it is your duty to empower your team by letting them handle their projects and tasks on their own. This technique also stimulates a sense of autonomy and promises professional advancement. For instance, If one of your team members does the work differently and creatively, he introduces creativity to the team. You must appreciate this innovation and creativity by rewarding that member for the idea.

You can also strengthen your team by introducing opportunities for career advancement. This proactive strategy will make your team members understand that the whole institution is interested in their long-term success.

The Basis of Positive Culture:

The bedrock of a positive work environment is trust. Nurse leaders cultivate and maintain a bond of trust through communication. They communicate openly and with transparency.

You can embed this practical strategy into your leadership journey by encouraging open communication. You can talk about realistic changes, challenges, goals, and limitations with your team members and hence, can succeed in building an environment based on trust and honesty. You will not only take the opinion or feedback of your team members while making a certain decision one time but will consider their opinions every time. Just like a dynamic leader, you will demonstrate reliability and responsibility by regularly following on through commitments and hence, building a culture based on dependability and reliability.

Forming and maintaining a healthy work environment in the field of nursing demands a set of proactive strategies. By forming a sense of belonging, encouraging constant improvements, promoting work-life balance, empowering teammates, and cultivating trust and reliability, you can ensure success on both individual and collective levels. Through these proactive techniques, you also embark on a journey that delivers the best patient care by winning fulfillment, commitment, and purpose in your professional life. In the evolving landscape of healthcare, these qualities become invaluable assets.

When talking about a positive work environment, the qualities of resilience and adaptability become the cornerstone of a successful leader. Therefore, it is important to learn how to embrace the wind of change as a leader.

Embracing Change as a Leader:

According to Orlin (2019), The Only Constant (in this world) is change. In the ever-changing field of nursing, change becomes the only constant. Nurse leaders must learn to navigate their staff successfully during the period of transformation. Let us continue to explore the benefits of communication, and resilience to embrace the changes in the healthcare community with the art of adaptability and grace.

Apprehending the Nature of Change in The Healthcare Institution:

As change is the only permanent reality within the walls of a healthcare system, it becomes important to learn about different forms of change. Change can come by wearing the cloak of new policies or wearing the mask of new technological equipment. You need to comprehend the nature of change within the healthcare ecosystem before implementing strategies to tackle these changes gracefully.

One way to address the change is via communicating the changes with your team effectively. As the protocols of change demand a change in attitude and old working style, communicating the change once might not be enough. Therefore, as a nurse leader, you will have to repeat the conversation a lot of times with your team, as repetition helps the mind to accept the change easily and quickly.

Make sure that you discuss the benefits and practices to overcome these challenges each time. As a productive outcome, you will notice that your team will have clarity about their goals and tasks and will be able to face these challenges easily.

Nurturing a Resilient Mindset:

The role of quality of resilience and adaptability has been emphasized a lot in the professional life of a nurse leader. It is time that we discuss resilience in detail. What exactly is resilience? How can you cultivate a resilient mindset?

The ability or the potential to bounce back from hurdles and obstacles is defined as resilience. It is the ability to adjust yourself to a change when things do not go the way you have planned that they will go. Likewise, a resilient mindset has the capacity and ability to recover quickly from challenges and difficulties without letting them affect your mental health. It does not mean that you cannot be upset, sad, or anxious; instead, it simply means that you do not let these emotions overcome your rationality and ability to overcome these challenges.

A resilient mind must be present in you and your team if you are planning to ascend the stairs of success together. As we all know, you will have to welcome the permanent face of change. Resilience can become your best friend in navigating the changes successfully.

When you are wearing the crown of nursing leadership, you become an ideal for your whole staff. They look at you and learn from you. As a nurse leader, it is your responsibility to choose to lead by good example. Let us imagine that during a time of change, your manager has advocated the importance of change in policies with its benefits, challenges, and goals effectively. You have understood the nature of change completely; however, you see that your boss is not following the protocols of the new policies. Will you be able to wear the uniform of resilience or choose to perform your day-to-day tasks as you used to before the change?

It is natural that you will choose the second option as you find the attitude of your boss unserious in the changing time. It is also possible that you will adopt new policies, but your performance will not be up to the mark as you are impacted by the example of your leader.

Now, envision the same scenario whenever you inform your team about the nature of change. Demonstrate resilience through your actions so that your team may learn from you. In addition to that, you can always share your personal experiences with your team so that they may adopt some proactive strategies to avoid hassle and difficulties during the change.

When sharing past experiences, you can also highlight those incidents when you and your team faced the challenging times of change successfully. The success stories from the past will offer them positivity, motivation, and strength to overcome these challenges.

Empowering Team Through Training:

When you have communicated the need for change and its impact on the healthcare system successfully, the next step is to talk about the set of skills and competencies needed to deal with the change.

You can facilitate your team by providing them with the necessary training to get the new skills needed. It is one of those times when you, as a nurse leader, will empower your team by offering them training- a chance to grow and flourish.

You can provide training through online resources, organizing workshops, and sharing worthy articles and practical examples. This way, you are not only empowering your team but also fostering a work culture that values adaptation and continuous learning.

To make the training programs more promising, you can also ask your team members to engage in the training to share their knowledge, insights, and skills. These training programs will help you create a collaborative work environment as well.

Recognizing Small Wins:

The worth of acknowledging and celebrating wins, no matter how small or large, grows more during times of change. The supportive and adaptive environment starts to flourish more as the celebrations result in boosting morale and maintaining success.

As a nurse leader, you can acknowledge the small steps of victory, as well as the efforts of your team members, even before embracing the final goal of success. When the final goal or the target has been met, you can implement a reward system to celebrate the moment of success.

The reward system can be of any type, including but not limited to recognition ceremonies, incentives, and chances of professional development.

In the changing world of nursing, the qualities of resilience and adaptability become a testament to the success that ensures that patient care remains the top priority in every phase of transformation.

Empowering Your Team:

> According to Maraboli (2014), "If you believe you can, you might. If you know you can, you will."

The definition of empowerment varies from person to person. However, it can be defined as the ability and practice to motivate and inform your actions, along with other peoples' actions, to embrace a particular mutual goal. Empowerment also means finding the power to not only motivate yourself but also take the initiative towards making decisions and achieving a particular target.

Empowerment in leadership is a transformative strategy that encompasses surpassing the boundaries of conventional hierarchical structures for the greater good, placing trust and autonomy in your team members. In the dynamic field of nursing, empowerment means equipping your team members with the necessary tools and confidence required to place themselves in an authoritative position. By putting themselves in the authoritative position, they will have more chances to contribute meaningfully to the overall success of the entire organization.

Empowerment is also an essential approach in practical leadership because it enhances job contentment, leads to innovation, and gives birth to efficiency in the healthcare industry.

Empowerment is synonymous with trust and as a nurse supervisor, you already have learned that you need to build trust within your team members. For example, you can demonstrate trust by showing your team members that you trust their abilities, have confidence in the power of their judgment, and feel that their commitment will help them to achieve mutual goals.

Hence, the key components of empowerment are trust, autonomy, delegation, and effective communication.

The Element of Trust:

Building a foundation of trust is fundamental to empowerment. You must trust your team members' abilities, judgment, and commitment to achieving shared goals.

The Power of Autonomy:

Empowerment also entails the act of providing individuals with the tool of autonomy. It also refers to making informed decisions all by yourself.

For example, you can give a level of autonomy to your team members by making them aware of their responsibilities. By knowing the scope of their responsibility, they will make good decisions that will contribute towards the success of the whole organization. The presence of autonomy also cultivates a sense of ownership and accountability among the team members.

The Act of Embracing Delegation:

A delegation is an act of distributing work among your team members by analyzing their skills and strengths.

As a nurse leader, you will find effective delegation as a cornerstone of the art of empowerment. You can assign tasks to each individual based on their skills, and development goals. Delegation welcomes success as it divides the tasks by analyzing the expertise of all individuals.

The Potential of Open Communication:

Empowerment can be demonstrated best through the use of open communication.

Being a nurse leader, you should engage in effective communication comprising of active listening, addressing concerns, and showing empathy.

Empathy is the art of understanding each other. As a nurse leader, you can show empathy by listening to your team members and implementing new policies by keeping in mind their concerns. We will talk more about empathy in the next chapters.

As we have talked about, the key components that build empowerment. Let us explore some of the benefits of empowerment.

Enhanced Job Satisfaction:

Empowered team members feel a heightened level of job fulfillment because they feel that they are valued and recognized for their contributions and efforts. They also recognize that their efforts are rewarding and they have a direct influence on the realm of patient care. This realization automatically enhances job satisfaction.

Increased Engagement and Motivation Rate:

The essence of empowerment lies in fueling motivation. When the staff feels trusted and experiences being the direct link between their efforts and healthy consequences, their engagement, as well as motivation, soar high in the sky.

Team Collaboration:

The team members feel that their efforts have a direct impact on the positive outcomes, and their leaders have guided them to form this connection. They start cultivating a workplace based on collaboration and a support system. This sense of collaborative spirit enhances the team's ability to overcome challenges easily.

Enhanced Problem-Solving Skills:

As empowerment is built from the bricks of autonomy, the empowered members of the team engage in innovative problem-solving skills, leading to the best decisions.

Let us have a glimpse at the abilities of an empowered team member. When the nurse, John feels empowered and knows that he has the freedom to express his ideas and plans and can afford to take risks, he automatically contributes to building a culture of improvements and adaptability. He brings this improvement via his problem-solving skills.

Higher Levels of Loyalty:

The role of empowered team members is not only to contribute to forming a positive work culture but also to enhance employment retention. When you make your team members feel appreciated, recognized, supported, and empowered, they reflect loyalty and try to continue to stick to their contributing role in impacting the whole organization.

Practical Strategies for Implementing Empowerment:

Let us embed the power of empowerment into your leadership so that you may enjoy the long-lasting perks of the power of empowerment.

As a nurse leader, you need to communicate your expectations, responsibilities, and goals effectively and clearly. When you communicate effectively, you gift your team members the ability to understand their roles, and they see how they can align their roles with broader team objectives.

You can invest in your team's advancement by providing continuous training and educational programs. Encourage them to participate in discussions and these training programs. Through continuous opportunities for growth, they will be able to enhance their efficiency in their current roles. Moreover, they will feel confident and will adapt better to future challenges and leadership roles.

The opportunities that you provide via learning and training will become the stepping stones to reach career advancement. You can also provide more opportunities by encouraging your team members to pursue education and certifications within the organization.

You can always encourage your staff to be involved in the decision-making process and take initiative for the well-being of the whole organization's success. You can also communicate the impact of opportunities in professional life.

As a nurse leader, you can also disclose your tale of success by narrating those incidents where you took risks synonymous with growth and learning opportunities.

When you celebrate small and large victories of your team or acknowledge the efforts of your team members, what you are doing is empowering your team. So, the seed of celebration grows in many branches, all aiming to achieve higher forms of success.

When you open the channel of transparent communication, make sure that you encourage the team members to offer their suggestions, feedback, and opinions in all matters. You must listen to each voice that offers valuable insights and fosters a culture of inclusivity and support.

You can also empower your team members by stepping into their shoes. For example, you can ask certain questions yourself, such as, what do you do when you feel entangled in a situation?

You might look for solutions by the technique of self-reflexivity or by seeking a mentor or a professional.

Become that mentor for your team so that they may come to you whenever they feel stranded in the web of difficulty and intricacy. Your effective mentorship will foster a professional relationship based on confidence and trust. They will appreciate your help by investing more time to achieve shared goals and tasks.

We all know that every benefit and success welcomes a myriad of challenges. Knowing these challenges beforehand can result in avoiding them altogether.

Let us have a look at all the faces of these hurdles in this effective leadership journey:

Resistance to Change:

Not everyone can welcome change optimistically, and it is fine as they feel afraid of change or sometimes lack the confidence to face it. These are the very reasons that power to empowerment comes into existence.

Whenever you feel that your team is resistant, you can always communicate with them. You can address their fears by discussing the benefits of the change and offer the necessary support and guidance during this transition.

Autonomy and Accountability:

When you provide the power of autonomy to your staff, it becomes challenging to ensure the balance between autonomy and accountability.

Being a leader, you can define clear expectations, monitor their progress, and offer useful feedback to balance this equilibrium.

Going ahead, we will dedicate more time to understanding how to balance autonomy and accountability.

Governing Diverse Perspectives:

When you empower your team to share opinions and participate in decision-making, dealing with various perspectives becomes quite difficult and challenging. You should fashion an inclusive, collaborative workplace environment by acknowledging all viewpoints and focusing on only those that lead to positive results.

Let us continue to empower ourselves by getting inspiration from a successful leader who empowered her team to achieve mutual goals of success.

Minu Mathew, one of the nurse leaders, met the challenges prevailing in her organization with the power of empowerment. She works in a care home, and when she started, she came to know that she needed the support of her team to perform well. As care home nursing is considered one of the most challenging areas in the world of healthcare organizations, some people believe that it is not technical at all because they find that the tasks are quite simple. However, Matthew reveals that the role is quite complicated as it involves a complete understanding of tasks and a full grip on knowledge and skills in the areas of care. As with any other profession, it demands commitment, passion, and hard work to perform the duties autonomously.

As a leader in a Teaching care home, she makes sure that the unregistered nurses who work with her are motivated, willing to learn more, and feel valued. Through her chain of efforts and empowerment, Mathews' team has helped her to touch the heights of individual and collective success (Contributor, 2017).

In conclusion, it is important to note that the journey to empower your team is more than a leadership technique; it is a transformational journey that fosters a workplace where your team members offer, support, and help each other to access the height of professional growth. Likewise, the collaborative environment reflects innovation and positivity.

By understanding the meaning of empowerment, along with its challenges and ways to overcome it, you, as a nurse leader, are ready to cultivate an environment where people will hear the echoes of long-term success.

Time For The Exercise:

- ↔ To empower your team members, you can arrange a virtual workshop where you will engage in exercises that inspire the team.

- For example, you can ask your team to brainstorm ideas and ways to justify the statement.

- "Shared Goals Fashion in Building a Sense of Purpose and Brings Unity Within the Team."

- Once they start to share their ideas and perspectives, encourage them by appreciating their efforts.

- You can also provide useful insights to justify the statement.

- Your engagement will motivate them to participate and take this exercise seriously.

After you have absorbed the principle of empowerment and proactive tactics, let us explore the halls of healthcare systems to unravel successful strategies so that you may advance in your professional career.

Chapter 5

Advancing Your Career in Nursing Leadership

One way to prepare yourself to deal with workplace issues is to learn how to deal with those issues. The other way to advance in your nursing career is to adopt effective career planning encompassing strong networking, and attaining leadership opportunities.

Let us scrutinize some of the best strategies for career planning, effective and strong networking and opportunities for practical leadership.

Strategic Career Planning:

The field of nursing is pregnant with a myriad of challenges ranging from a shortage of staff to implementing changing healthcare policies. All such issues can be addressed and tackled proactively in the landscape of strategic career planning, which also helps score professional and organizational success.

Self-evaluation is the key to effective career planning. You will have to constantly evaluate your set of expertise, areas for improvement, strengths, and weaknesses. For instance, by evaluating your set of skills consisting of weaknesses and strengths, you will come to know that you lack improved communication skills. After identifying the area of improvement, you can engage in ways to overcome your obstacle. This gap can be filled by attending training programs, engaging in conversation with your fellows, and seeking guidance from your mentors.

As we have already understood the importance of networking, it is still important to mention the power of networking to pave a path towards success seamlessly and proactively. Building connections from the very start of your profession will open the doors of vast seas of knowledge and actionable strategies during uncertain and challenging times.

Fashioning your professional image is an integral part of career planning. You can always create your positive professional image through online platforms, including but not limited to Facebook, LinkedIn, and other various social websites. The process of building your professional image also goes through the room of your achievements and distinctions.

In the demanding and changing field of nursing, the role of contribution to your industry is of immense importance. Let us understand it through a simple example. When you go to a shopping mall to buy, the salesperson asks for the specifications and then finds the one suitable for you. Now, step into the shoes of a salesperson. When you are planning to get a promotion or advancement in your career, you will need to show your worth through your skills and your contributions to your industry so that they may know that you are suitable for that particular role. Now, you can enjoy the success.

Education and degrees are also part of effective strategic career planning. Pursuing advanced degrees, certificates, and diplomas and attending workshops can also guarantee career success as they show commitment to the profession and help overcome shortcomings. Meet Nurse Lowen, who found that she was lacking in decision-making and problem-solving skills. Therefore, her aspiration is to achieve a certification in healthcare management. As a result, she has become proficient in decision-making abilities. She is more confident that she will succeed in her profession of nursing leadership.

A nurse leader always knows what she wants and what her aspirations are. Therefore, you need to align your personal goals with your organization's mission and start working to attain long-term objectives. This timely alignment will also hone your other skills like time management because you have started to work on attaining long-term goals in a set period of time. For example, a nurse leader observed the need for new patient care initiatives as soon as possible in the healthcare unit. She started planning the execution in a set time frame. The execution honed her skills in problem-solving and time management as well.

Nursing leadership is about continuous and sustainable efforts to maintain the sustainability of their teams. By participating in succession planning, you can ensure the sustainable success of your workforce. By identifying the leadership potential in the team, the cycle of sustainable success can be maintained effectively. Besides that, it also helps prepare the team for future challenges. You can mentor and assist one of your skilled staff members by providing guidance and roads full of opportunities for the role of leader.

You can adopt the strategy of *SMART* goals: Specific, Measurable, Achievable, Relevant, and Time-Bound to advance in your career as well.

S-M-A-R-T:

An unclear destination plan leads to futile wandering. If you define and see a clear picture of your career goals, you can achieve them more easily and timely. You can start by specifying a particular destination, such as, "Earn a Nurse Leadership Role in the Care unit by 2025", rather than setting a generalized aim like " Get Success In my career."

The specific aim has set your mind to achieve one particular goal and to align your skills that lead to the accomplishment of that skill.

Now that you have mastered the *specific* part of SMART. Let us move on to the *measurable* part. When you set a lot of ambitions and goals, measurable ones start to navigate your course. For instance, if you aim to "Enhance patient satisfaction by 20% in the time period of seven months," you will achieve that part of the goal easily. Why? The reason is simple, actually. Your measurable quantity has broken down the criteria of success into tangible and short-term goals. When you fulfill them, you start to feel satisfied and more confident. However, if you plan to "increase patient care" simply, you work harder without getting the best result. It is because without any measurable goal, you will remain unsatisfied, and the more you work, the more you will think that you have achieved nothing much.

One of the most impactful strengths in the course of your destination is the *achievability* of your goals and tasks. You can achieve a goal if it is based on reality and can be clutched through a realistic approach. It does not mean that you cannot think about revolutionizing or introducing a new form in your healthcare environment; instead, it simply means that such a road to success is paved only when you have achieved a set of more realistic achievements and have a realistic approach towards this goal in your career. Rather than focusing on a goal like "Revolutionize the healthcare institutions globally," please form a goal like "Get the certificate in Advanced Cardiovascular Life Support this year." This realistic goal will compel you to move steadily toward your goal.

You can also align your career vision with some *relevant* aims that will help you achieve your main goal. It is like embodying the principles of effective communication in your personal life so that it may help you when you become a democratic leader. Similarly, if you want to become a nurse leader, you may align your relevant goal, that is, "polish leadership skills by attending and participating in the management workshop within the next three months."

When you are setting specific, measurable, achievable, and relevant goals, you are also setting a limit by which you have to achieve those goals. In simple words, that limit or boundary is time. You might be wondering what happens when you set a time limit.

When you envision a goal by specifying a *time* limit, you are actually preparing your mind to start working immediately to achieve that specific goal.

SMART is not only about giving yourself a clear goal but also a clear time frame.

Effective career planning is a phenomenon of periodic evaluation. Therefore, you need to assess your goals and aspirations and change your course of action constantly. Constant evaluation ensures evolution in your career development as well.

In essence, effective career planning is an intentional process that empowers you to take charge of your professional destinies.

You can always take help from your personalized roadmap by looking at your long-term as well as short-term goals.

Effective Networking for Leadership Success:

We have already discussed a little bit about the value of effective networking necessary for leadership success. Let us unravel its whole potential for leadership success.

When you are trying to build a successful network, you are always advised to form a sound network. This sound networking helps in ensuring successful leadership. Therefore, you need to accumulate those people whose values align with your own and who believe in the power of growing and advancing together. Prioritize the quality of people over the number of people. In simple words, you need to build deep and meaningful relationships.

There are many ways to build a strong network:

Professional Associations:

You can form effective networking by participating in professional organizations. You can join and engage in leadership associations or organizations that help you advance in your career. You can also attend conferences, workshops, seminars, and such occasions to connect with people who have the same goals as you. They can also offer useful insights to help you in difficult times.

Build an Online Presence:

Fortify your connection further by engaging your colleagues and like-minded people through online platforms. This will unburden you to attend or join a program in a specific setting.

Seek Mentorship:

When you come across healthcare industry leaders and professionals, you can seek for mentorship. These mentors will not only guide you but also help you expand your network through their own connections.

Invest Time Carefully:

As networking is an ongoing process of fostering professional relationships, please be careful and intentional, for you are investing your time in people.

Building such connections does not mean using people for your own benefit only. Instead, it is about forming deep relationships where you feel yourself ready to help them as well.

Collaborate:

Collaborating with the people in your organization and other healthcare community can open the door to forming meaningful relationships. When working together during a project or for an organization, you can also create network opportunities through teamwork.

Leadership Development Programs:

You can also join several leadership development programs that enhance leadership skills. These platforms not only hone your leadership skills but also connect you with people who are trying to become leaders, just like you.

The Art of Words:

Effective networking stems from effective communication. When you have to introduce yourself in any meeting, seminar, or professional setting, introduce yourself in a compelling manner by talking about your current role and your expected role as a nurse leader in the future. This concise introduction will help you form a network in such a professional setting.

As your goal is to find people with similar aspirations like you, listen actively when others speak. Show genuine interest in others' perspectives, and you will see that it has established a good rapport. Your serious attitude will set you as a person who values knowledge and a collaborative environment.

Once you have found a connection with people due to these events and organizations, contact them regularly to maintain the networking. You can send them messages reflecting your appreciation for the effective interaction. You can also talk about mutual opportunities where you can stay connected.

Equal Reciprocity: Give and Receive

Effective networking is bidirectional (two-way street). When you are looking for help and guidance, be open to offering assistance and guidance to others. You can offer your knowledge, insights, and pieces of advice to other members of the same community as well. This positions you as an invaluable asset in the professional realm.

One way to make this two-way street effective is by facilitating introductions. For instance, In your network, if you recognize collaboration opportunities between members, you can facilitate introductions. Your role as a connector will strengthen your network and will earn you a reputation for being someone who believes in contributing to the growth of other fellows.

When you receive support and assistance from professionals and mentors, you need to show gratitude through messages or by contributing to the whole organization by supporting others. Your display of gratitude forms a positive and healthy network culture where your connections feel valued and respected.

Through this, you are also fostering a mindset of reciprocity to form mutually advantageous relationships.

Evaluate Your Impact:

When you are moving forward, it is necessary to take a moment to look back to appreciate small wins and consequences. Likewise, when you have built the network, do not forget to ponder upon the impacts of your efforts. For example, you can look at the quality of the relationships you have cultivated, the insights you have learned, and the opportunities that you have earned through your network.

You can also evaluate how much your network has assisted you in attaining professional growth from time to time. You can ask these questions for evaluation:

- Have I gained new insights?

- Have I gathered some valuable knowledge?

- Did I find any opportunity that aligns with my career objectives?

- Did I access all these opportunities that lead to career advancement?

- When you are evaluating the impact of your network, you also need to reflect on the depth of your relationships. You can ask yourself the questions like :

- Have I fostered meaningful connections that surpass the trajectory of professional niceties?

Sometimes, good professional relationships lead to fostering professional partnerships.

As your dream is career advancement in the ever-evolving field of nursing, reflect if your network has the capability to guide you through the changing times in your professional journey. Align your network in accordance with your long-term objectives.

Navigating Leadership Opportunities:

The nurses have the potential to transform themselves into influential nurse leaders by identifying career growth opportunities and getting benefits from them.

Directing Quality Improvement Ambitions:

In most of the healthcare institutions, qualitative improvement has become a permanent endeavor. Nurses can engage in the role of nurse leader by actively participating in quality improvement initiatives.

For example, you notice a recurring challenge occurring while handling patient care handovers.

You and your colleagues have reported the issue a lot of times. However, no improvement can be seen. What should you do in such a situation?

You can choose to wear the cloak of a leader and can lead by implementing a more efficient handover process. You can also reduce errors and faults to improve patient outcomes.

> **Key Takeaway:** You have seized an opportunity to enhance quality improvement that demonstrates a proactive leadership approach.

Mentoring Junior Members:

You can contribute to the growth of individuals, teams, and the entire organization through the art of mentorship.

Imagine that a new nurse has joined your team, and she has a lot of potential, but it is misdirected. You can take the role of a mentor by offering guidance and sharing useful insights. Through this leadership role, you have successfully contributed to the unit's educational culture of constant growth.

> **Key Takeaway:** The proactive leadership role has given you the authority to lead a team and build a network.

Engaging In Collaboration:

In the intricate world of the healthcare industry, interdisciplinary collaboration is of prime importance. Nurse fellows can engage and participate in interdisciplinary committees and take the lead.

Imagine: In the bustling halls of your healthcare community, the process of patient care varies from unit to unit. These different approaches result in delayed actions and unsatisfactory patient satisfaction rates.

You want to enhance the patient rate by following the same instructions. How can you convince all the disciplines to follow one specific approach?

You can organize regular meetings on the subject of a collective approach to patient care so that all professionals from various departments and disciplines may join it.

These meetings will not only improve your patient satisfaction rate but also enhance your communication skills.

> **Key Takeaway:** Adopting an interdisciplinary collaboration approach gives you the opportunity to become a leader who values coordinated patient care.

Seizing Opportunities Exceeding Your Existing Position:

When you dream of becoming a nurse leader, it is important for you to seize opportunities that go beyond your current role. It can be done in multiple ways:

Enhancing and refining skills through advanced certifications is one of the best strategic moves that invites multiple opportunities for the role of nurse leader.

For example, if you are passionate about oncology nursing, you can earn an Oncology Certified Nurse (OCN) certificate. This OCN certification will not only help you deepen your strengths and skills but also multiply your chances to pursue your leadership role, either in collaborative leadership or contributing to industry development.

You can also showcase your acquired leadership skills by volunteering for special projects. For example, you notice that there is a gap in patient educational materials, and you want to modify the educational material. So, you can take a lead in the educational resources that are comprehensive and complete.

Whether you have pursued a certificate in professional nursing or choose to volunteer to lead a particular project, you are demonstrating active involvement. Active involvement is one of the main needs of the demanding field of nursing. Hence, this engagement and involvement will make it easy for you to achieve your goals.

You can also access other leadership development programs by getting involved in other organizations, such as the American Nurses Association (ANA) or the Sigma Theta Tau International Honor Society of Nursing. These organizations will help you to establish more networks.

> **Key Takeaway:** Pursuing advanced certifications reflects your commitment to excellence by paving a path toward leadership positions in specialized areas.

Now that we have learned to navigate leadership opportunities let us try to enhance our decision-making skills through some of the exercises:

Exercise 01:

During shift hangovers in a bustling medical-surgical unit, you observed a pattern of medication errors multiple times. You have the option to report the issue immediately. However, you choose to seize the opportunity to show your leadership skills.

- How will you execute your leadership skills in an effective way?

- Think about it for some time!

You, along with, a team of nurses may choose to implement the handover phenomenon, organize training sessions, and introduce a system of checklist. The outcome can be remarkable: a significant reduction in medication errors and also mirrors your compassionate side by highlighting your commitment to patient safety.

Exercise 02:

When working in a critical care unit, you recognized communication issues between the members of the nursing and respiratory therapy teams.

- How can you turn this issue into an opportunity to show your leadership role?
- Envision a solution!

You can take the initiative by organizing regular interdisciplinary meetings to discuss the ways to improve patient care mutually. In those meetings, share knowledge and encourage others to do so. It will help you start a unified communication within all teams. This will help you to improve your leadership skills by focusing on teamwork.

Exercise 03:

You pursue a certification in Maternal Newborn Nurse (RNC-MNN) as you feel devoted to maternal health.

- How is this degree helping you to pave a path toward successful leadership?
- You can think about some emergency situations!

Your knowledge after pursuing advanced certifications has been enhanced, and your skills have been further polished. In the delivery unit, your certificate has positioned you as a go-to resource. In simple words, your skills have contributed to the formation of evidence-based practices in the unit.

In conclusion, seizing leadership opportunities demands a blend of awareness, initiative, and critical decision-making. Besides this, quality improvement initiatives, attaining advanced education, or arranging a collaborative meeting can lead nurses toward success.

Time for The Excercise:

- ↝ Envision your career aspirations by closing your eyes.

- ↝ Feel the warmth after you have embraced the success in your nursing leadership journey.

- ↝ Now, it is time to create a vision board.

- ↝ Write or attach pictures of your success and goals.

- ↝ This Vision Board is your reminder to keep on moving forward until you embrace success.

The goal is to make your vision a reality: "If my mind can conceive it, and my heart can believe it - then I can achieve it (Ali, 2013)."

As you have planned your career progression strategically, you are not only getting a step closer to your success but also sculpting your legacy of being a successful nurse leader. In the next chapter, we will examine the transformative journey so far and focus on the significance of continuous growth in the dynamic field of nursing leadership.

So, let us embark on a new chapter of a successful journey toward leadership, where we will travel through strategic avenues to explore the profound impact of your leadership journey.

Share Your Thoughts!

Hello Readers,

Hope you're doing great! We're excited to hear what you think about the book "Empower Your Nursing Leadership" by Brandy Covington. This book is all about helping nurses become awesome leaders!

Your opinion is super important, especially because you're a leader in the world of nursing. Your thoughts can help other nurses decide if this book is right for them.

Can you tell us:

What you liked: Did you find cool stuff in the book that you can use in your nursing leader journey?

How it helps you: Were you able to use what you read in the book in your everyday nursing leader life? Can you give examples?

What you learned: Did the book teach you new things about being a leader in nursing? Did it change the way you think about leading?

We're so curious to know how this book made a difference for you. Your thoughts can help other nurses, too!

You can send your review by clicking [website link]. If you have any questions, ask away!

Thanks a bunch for being awesome in the world of nursing. We can't wait to hear what you think about "Empower Your Nursing Leadership."

Cheers,

Brandy Covington

Chapter 6

Reflecting on Your Leadership Journey

In the advancing world of nursing leadership, sparing some time to reflect on your journey so far becomes one of the powerful tools for growth. As a leader, You will have to learn from only those experiences that can lead to professional growth.

Let us learn the transformative power of the art of self-reflection to continue climbing the ladder of leadership growth and advancement.

The Art of Self-Reflection:

Self-reflection is also known as personal reflection. It refers to the act of taking the time to think about, meditate, assess, and ponder upon your behaviors, thoughts, aptitudes, set of motivations, and desires. It is a phenomenon of digging deep into the trove of your thoughts, ideas, and emotions to find out the reason or the answer to the 'why' hidden beneath them.

Therefore, in your leadership journey, the art of self-reflection is a very useful tool as it aims for professional development by promoting awareness regarding your (previous) actions.

In this explorative journey, we will dive into the significance of self-reflection and unravel some of its powerful techniques like introspection and journaling, that can cultivate a reflective and progressive mindset successfully.

Benefits of Self-Reflection:

Through proactive strategies that teach us the ways to change the hurdles into growth opportunities, we all acknowledge that leadership is not all about showing your managing skills (managing others); it is also about managing and supervising yourself. Through self-reflection, you can learn about your strengths, flaws, beliefs, values, goals, and motivations. By using the technique of self-reflection that allows you to gain insight into your thoughts through problem-solving, analysis, journalling, mindfulness, or introspection. Listed below are some of the answers to 'whys.' Self-reflection is an essential tool in the society of leadership.

Enriched Self-Awareness:

Self-awareness is the experience of having an utter understanding of your personality, encompassing your thoughts, emotions, values, aspirations, beliefs, and actions. That is the reason that self-awareness is the bedrock of effective and powerful leadership.

As a self-reflective nurse leader, you can make good decisions that will cater to your values by understanding your own actions, reactions, emotions, and thought patterns.

Enriched Decision-Making Skill:

The process of understanding your values, strengths, weaknesses, actions, and emotions is by analyzing your experiences, past choices, and their consequences. The time you invest in self-reflection, especially delving into your past, may seem futile or overwhelming to you at first, but this feeling will not be a permanent one. Gradually, you will be able to use the tools of past experiences to enhance your decision-making skills.

After analyzing, you will be able to identify your mistakes, learn from them, and hence make good and informed decisions.

Influential Communication:

When you are analyzing your past and the choices you made back then, you are continuously involved in the act of communication with yourself. Therefore, the leaders who are involved in the art of self-reflection are more attuned to their communication styles.

Their communication style varies from situation to situation, echoes with diverse audiences, and cultivates better understanding within the spheres of their teams.

Through this effective communication with yourself, you will also be able to adapt to different styles of communication.

Adaptability and Education:

The cloak of adaptability is significant in the landscape of successful leadership. This technique can be learned through the skill of self-reflection. This skill enables you to learn from your past, invest in your present situation, and align your actions with future goals. All these actions and seeds of knowledge teach you the art of adaptability as well.

Let us learn how to implement the techniques of self-reflection into our professional lives.

Techniques for Self-Reflection:

Introspection:

One of the best ways to get in touch with your inner thoughts is through introspection. It encompasses a deep understanding of your thoughts, emotions, and experiences.

Introspection will help you foster a deeper and clearer understanding of yourself.

You can engage in this activity by setting a time dedicated to this activity every day. In that dedicated time, you can meditate on certain scenarios and circumstances, by taking into account the resulting emotional responses and then finding reasons for their responses. If you find out that those contributing factors are beneficial, you can implement those factors to drive the desired outcomes in challenging situations.

Mindfulness:

Mindfulness simply is the state of being aware of yourself. Mindfulness practices can be adopted in your life through the art of meditation and the rhythmic heartbeat of mindful breathing.

As a leader, you will be able to understand your thoughts without any clouds of judgment. Besides this, it will promote clarity and transparency and bring focus. You will get a lot of benefits through mindfulness in high-pressure situations. These high-pressure situations can range from making swift decisions during challenging times to introducing a new policy within a set time period.

Journaling:

Jotting down your thoughts is one of the easiest and most useful ways to clear your head from the noisy clutter of thoughts. You can always write about your experiences along with their consequences. You can also talk about the lessons you have learned from these experiences.

It is important to talk about the lessons as it will keep your mind focused in a productive direction.

When you have to face a hurdle in your leadership journey, you can review these written experiences and form a resolution in time.

Feedback :

When you are writing about the consequences of your choices, you are both analyzing your chain of actions and the reactions of the people around you. Sometimes, the reaction of the people (written, communication, or impressions) becomes one of the most important parts in helping you form sound decisions in the future.

This act of analyzing other people's reactions is simply valuing the feedback received from your colleagues, mentors, and juniors. The optimistic feedback, along with diverse perspectives, will help you understand more about your leadership style and its influence on others.

How To Cultivate a Reflective Mindset:

Create Time for Reflection:

The art of self-reflection becomes beneficial through the act of repetition.

As a leader, it becomes difficult to find some time to reflect; however, it does not mean that we can skip it. You can always start through small steps.

For instance, you can carve out only a few minutes dedicated to mindfulness each morning. If that is not suitable, you can also try journaling once a week.

No one knows the worth of consistency, dedication, and patience more than a nursing leader who is serving a dynamic healthcare community.

Embrace Vulnerability:

As a reflective leader, you will not only identify your mistakes but also embrace them. Embracing vulnerability will help you develop a workplace based on openness, honesty, and trust. Likewise, your actions will inspire and empower other peers to engage in the practice of self-reflection.

Set Goals for Growth:

As self-reflection helps you understand yourself, it also improves your professional life and impacts your personal life in the best manner. But do you wonder what will happen if you intentionally align your professional and personal growth aspirations with the art of self-reflection?

You will enjoy quick progress in both aspects of life.

You can also keep track of the success of your self-reflection by observing the progress over time.

Incorporate Reflection into Leadership Development Programs:

As a leader, you are not only responsible for managing your success but also contributing toward the development of the whole community. You can incorporate the essential components of self-reflection into your leadership training and development programs. You can also suggest your organizations include introspection in their training and educational programs.

Ostensibly, the practice of self-reflection is one of the transformative approaches in the dynamic world of leadership. It asserts that the journey toward the outer and external success comes from the journey within.

Learning from Challenges and Successes:

When you have to learn from your past, you have to visit the tunnels of time, and it can be exhausting. You can overlook a mistake or forget to learn from your success, therefore, it is necessary to learn how to understand and identify those challenges that lead to your success in your leadership career.

Let us reflect upon the usual kinds of challenges that you may have encountered or will encounter in your leadership career. You will also learn how to learn from these experiences.

Staffing Shortages:

One of the most persistent challenges you will encounter in your leadership journey will be navigating a staff shortage. You will have to balance the needs of your patients with the limited available resources. Therefore, it becomes quite challenging to maintain a balance with the needs of the patient simultaneously.

You can find a solution through strategic thinking and resilience.

Now, revise what you have learned from this challenge.

You might have learned that such a challenge can be tackled by creative problem-solving (strategic thinking), building the morale of your team through effective communication, and the significance of your delegation.

Communication Breakdowns:

In your healthcare industry, you might have gone through a time when you saw that fragmented communication has led to critical issues such as working together for a shared goal. Your manager did not provide you with enough information, and so you communicated only half of the details.

How can you learn to tackle this challenge?

Through self-reflection, you will find out that effective and clear communication helps enhance the whole team's effectiveness and efficiency and fosters a collaborative system.

Likewise, through self-reflection, you might have come to the fact that listening actively and constructive feedback can lead to forming strong communication strategies that lead to successful leadership advancement.

Adapting to Change:

As change is the only permanent reality in the evolving land of the healthcare industry, therefore, you might have faced this issue. Be it the challenge of Implementing new technologies or introducing new policies, you might have worn the coat of adaptability and flexibility.

Through this challenge, you might have learned that:

Facing the change with a positive set of attitude and mindset can help you a lot. Besides this, as the leader, you have to always empower and guide your team members through the tool of effective communication.

Balancing Compassion and Professionalism:

When you see a lot of patients depend upon you for care and the touch of healing, you not only feel compassion, but sometimes, you feel overwhelming emotions. It is one of the by-products of being in the profession of healthcare.

You might have gone through this issue, especially at the start of your career. You might have cultivated a balance between compassion for your patients and maintaining a professional attitude all the way long. Through the strategy of effective emotional intelligence, you might have overcome this dilemma.

You learned from this experience that:

You can always offer the best and top-notch patient care while feeling compassionate for the patient; however, it is not in your hands to recover them quickly and as per their expectations. You might have learned that writing about these overwhelming feelings and sentiments or sharing these emotions with someone can be really helpful for your health.

Now that we have looked into the benefits of the challenges let us have a glimpse of your success that can also teach you a lot of things.

Team Unity:

In your leadership journey, you might have been able to use your effective communication skills to bring your team together. This would have resulted in a huge success.

What can you learn from this successful event in your career?

You learned that maintaining a collaborative team network has multiplied the score of success. Similarly, it has cultivated a work environment where harmony, trust, and support resonate with the actions of the people.

Also, you noticed that your team members feel valued, and therefore, they invest their effort in achieving a goal and enjoy the process all along.

Patient-Centered Care Initiatives:

As a nurse leader, you saw that patient care is not satisfactory. Therefore, you offered some patient care initiatives that led to an enhanced rate of patient satisfaction.

What insights did you get from this particular success story?

You might have learned that enhancing patients' experiences has resulted in enhanced quality of patient care that has increased the patient satisfaction rate. You also might have observed that the initiatives have empowered your team as they involve the blend of empathy and education.

Professional Development:

In the nursing world, there are many opportunities in the form of training and mentorship workshops. These opportunities might have knocked on the door of your professional life. You seized the opportunity, and now you have become a more successful leader.

What did you learn from this experience?

You observed that engaging in these workshops has boosted your confidence. It has allowed you to contribute to the professional growth of your team members. Through this, you have also fostered a workplace that values continuous learning.

Effective Crisis Management:

You were navigating successfully through the stability of time; however, over time, things started to take a turn. To maintain success, you made a swift decision and boosted the morale of your team, which resulted in achieving your targets.

What is it about the experience that will stay with you always?

You might have learned that adaptability, effective communication, and preparedness lead to long-term success in the long haul of both personal and professional phases of life.

Through the art of reflection, you have noticed that the path to your successful leadership journey has passed through the lands of failures and successes. Both have fortified your leadership spirit, and in the future, it will do the same.

In the future, when you come across these circumstances or similar ones, you will know what to do, and it will save you time as well. You can look into the notebook of self-reflection to find a more refined answer.

Feedback as a Catalyst for Improvement:

We have talked about the importance of feedback time and again. Let us discuss it in detail to know more about it.

One of the powerful tools in fostering a positive environment is feedback. As a nurse leader, it can serve as a mirror for you, reflecting your weaknesses and strengths.

Therefore, it is very crucial to apply positive and constructive feedback to enhance efficient leadership.

Let us now explore the significance of feedback:

As feedback serves as a mirror, you can look into it to learn about your leadership style, identify your strengths, highlight your weaknesses, and find areas for improvement.

In essence, it becomes a stimulus and catalyst for growth, and at the same time, it also brings self-awareness and enables you as a leader to formulate your actions in accordance with your intentions, goals, and values.

When you provide feedback or give a rating to a product that you bought. You intend to say what you feel about the product honestly. Moreover, if there is room for improvement in this product, you expect them to take the review, rating, or feedback professionally and with the intention to improve it.

When you get feedback from your mentors or staff members, adopt the same mindset. As a leader, you can see it as an opportunity for growth that will foster your abilities through the foundations of dedication and hard work.

Just like effective communication, feedback is a two-way street. You should not only ask for input from your team members constantly, but you should also fashion an environment where you can provide honest and constructive feedback to your staff by evaluating their performance. This will help you build an environment based on open communication and trust. This constructive approach will contribute to the collective success of your team.

Requesting Constructive Feedback:

As a nurse leader, you can foster a culture where you can demonstrate that the feedback is not only accepted but also encouraged. You can tell your team members that feedback is not about judgment, it is about improvement.

When someone gives you feedback, like communicate effectively about the limitations of a sudden change. You should appreciate them and should look for strategies to succeed in your professional life.

Next time, when they see that their feedback has been taken constructively, they will reciprocate. It is called leading by example.

Regular Check-Ins:

You can schedule regular check-ins with your staff to talk about their perspectives on your leadership. You can employ open-ended questions to drive meaningful discussions about support, change, and chances for professional development. These constant check-ins cultivate a consistent loop of feedback that ensures timely adjustments and improvements.

Anonymous Feedback Process:

Sometimes, the staff members hesitate to provide feedback directly for many reasons. As a nurse leader, you can ensure that everyone should share their feedback by remaining in their safe space. You can conduct anonymous surveys or offer suggestion boxes to gather honest feedback by eliminating the feelings of fear of reprisal.

This feedback approach also appreciates open communication and ensures that all the diverse voices are heard.

360-Degree Feedback:

You can gather feedback from various sources, including but not limited to colleagues, professionals, and mentors. A 360-degree feedback phenomenon offers a complete insight into your leadership influence. This well-rounded feedback can unravel spots that offer a more holistic understanding of your distinctive leadership style.

Utilizing Feedback for Skill Improvement:

Active Listening:

As a nurse leader, when you are receiving feedback, exercise the skill of active listening.

If you think that your intention or goal has been misunderstood, you can always try to communicate it effectively. Rather than becoming defensive, shift your focus to understand the shared perspectives thoroughly. After the feedback, express gratitude by telling them how significant their role is in the field of self-improvement. It will position you as someone who values commitment and continuous learning.

Set Clear Goals for Improvement:

When you have received the feedback, set your new goals clearly. As you have identified your areas of improvement, start working on them accordingly. You can break down these aims into smaller steps so that you may implement these changes effectively,

Remember that the key to growth is consistency. You can always evaluate your progress and make adjustments as well.

Feedback Is a Learning Opportunity:

Instead of seeing feedback as an obstacle or a shortcoming, learn from it and see it as an opportunity to grow and evolve. You can access each piece of feedback with an air of curiosity and desire to grow.

Time For the Excercise:

- Start writing about your experiences and challenges in a journal.

- You can call it a Leadership Journal.

- Jote down every significant emotion, value, and aspiration that you went through in your professional life.

- Now, align those emotions and aspirations with your professional growth.

- Whenever you encounter a similar situation, look back into your journal and take a lead in your successful leadership career.

Self-reflection is not a pause in your career growth; it is an act of contact learning and moving toward success. So, do not let the thought cross your mind that you are embarking on your journey to the past; rather, you are moving strategically toward the future.

In the next chapter, we will delve into the influence and impact of nursing leadership in the spheres of the healthcare community and the well-being of the whole organization.

Chapter 7

Fostering Positive Work Environments in Nursing Leadership

Be it the art of self-reflection, dealing with challenges, or acquiring a successful nursing leadership career, we keep on talking about the cultivation of a positive work environment.

Why does a positive workplace hold this much importance?

Imagine that, being a nurse manager, you have facilitated your staff with a flexible schedule, communicated about new challenges effectively, and informed them about the impact of new goals. Through your efforts, your team has not only learned about their role but also acknowledged their contribution to the healthcare community. They will start working in one unified direction that will lead to accumulative success.

However, if you have noticed the germ of non-healthy competition in your team and you mistake it for more productivity and more success. What will be the outcomes?

Will the guards of healthcare facilities guide each other in challenging times? Will they be able to breathe peacefully, unaffected by the burdens of toxicity, while performing their duties? Obviously not. Purports that in a workplace where positivity, well-being, and support resonate, both individual and collective success thrives.

As a nurse leader, you have a direct and indirect role in shaping your work environment on the foundations of positivity and collaboration. Therefore, we will discover some of the most significant strategies that can help you foster a healthy workplace.

Prioritizing Staff Well-being:

We have already talked about your well-being in the previous chapters. In this section, we will talk about your role as a nurse leader to guide your team members regarding their health and well-being.

In the realm of nursing leadership, the easiest way to impact your surroundings is through leading by example: prioritize your health, take care of your mental peace, restore your mental energy by taking breaks, and enjoy your free time.

In order to enhance job satisfaction and organizational performance, it is important that you build a positive work setting. In your leadership journey, you can implement strategies and factors, from mental health to stress management, that can enhance job satisfaction.

Let us explore some of the best factors and strategies that contribute to a positive workplace.

Work-Life Balance:

As a nurse leader, you have experienced that the workload in the nursing field is quite exhausting, and if it can be exhausting for you, it will be exhausting and frustrating for your team members, especially for juniors who have to adapt to the environment. Therefore, you should start your training by asserting the importance of work-life balance.

You can make your staff aware of the importance by asserting that excessive workload and long working hours without any breaks will lead to burnout, heavy stress, and dissatisfaction. The outcome of the effects will be that they will not be able to perform well. Nurse managers should also guide their staff to work on reasonable work hours, discourage the culture of overwork, and offer flexible working schedules when needed or whenever possible.

Through these guidelines, you will be able to increase your level of productivity, and your employees will feel more focused and motivated during their working hours.

Professional Growth Opportunities:

When the members of your healthcare facility see the constant opportunities for growth and advancement, they do not feel stuck in a position for a longer period. They try to succeed in their professional lives by performing well. This phenomenon keeps the nursing ecosystem dynamic and evolving.

When you give them the chance to grow, they feel that their skills are being acknowledged and that there is room for growth. They will become more engaged, mentally peaceful, and dedicated to their roles.

As a nurse leader, you can take the initiative by asking your organization to invest in training programs, mentorship conferences, or workshops, as it will teach your team how to benefit from these opportunities.

Communication and Transparency:

You can also promote a culture of open communication within your unit. It will build trust. Additionally, whenever your employees feel that they are not satisfied with their working schedule or it is affecting their health, they will prefer to come to talk to you.

Likewise, you can reach out to your employees if you feel that their performance is being affected for some reason. By knowing the contributing factors, you can guide them on how to tackle them.

For example, If the reason lies that they are working constantly without any break. You can ask them to take breaks regularly. Moreover, you need to guide them in the fact that it is essential for their health to take regular breaks.

As a nurse leader, you have the power to organize meetings and seminars where you will empower your team members and other professionals to share their insights on the importance of well-being.

When you are organizing seminars and conducting workshops in your workplace, you can talk about various topics. Additionally, you can launch programs, including fitness programs, stress management classes, encouraging access to counseling services, and publishing articles on the side effects of excessive burns.

By establishing a culture where health is as important as the work, you are empowering your staff to take care of themselves at every level.

Employee Assistance Programs (EAPs):

In EAPs, you can support and guide your staff when they face a clash between their personal and professional levels. Employee assistance programs usually provide counseling, mental health services, and ways to tackle personal issues so that an individual may work efficiently.

Through EAPs, you can not only foster a culture of supportive work environment but position yourself as someone who values the wellbeing of their staff just as you value yours.

In a work environment, cultivating a system of recognition and reward can both boost morale and enhance job satisfaction. Besides introducing incentives, monthly rewards, and certificates of acknowledgment, you can adopt certain strategies to foster a system of collective mental well-being. You can also introduce rewards for the employee of the month so that the reward ceremonies may become habitual.

Let us discuss the importance of establishing a culture of acknowledgment and appreciation.

Building a Culture of Appreciation:

In the world of healthcare, nurses usually work in intense, emotionally charged, and physically challenging environments. In such a world, the culture of appreciation can rejuvenate their mental happiness and dignity.

As a nurse leader, tokens of professional appreciation and admiration should be an integral part of your responsibilities. When appreciating your staff, you must maintain a thin line of balance between productive and non-productive appreciation.

Productive appreciation is the one where your staff will know that they are being valued and they are getting the reward for their efforts. Therefore, it will motivate and inspire them to work more vigilantly and cheerfully. In addition to that, they will know that their consistent dedication is the key to unlocking a door of accomplishments.

You can also empower your team by expressing words of appreciation and acknowledgment regularly. You can foster a custom of regular appreciation and celebration by implementing any of these strategies:

Peer-to-Peer Recognition Programs:

When you are stressed about the outcomes of your dauntless efforts, kind words of appreciation from your fellows can boost your morale. You also get a positive sense of direction that helps you invest your time and efforts more productively.

Envision this scenario within your healthcare unit. As a nurse leader, you have the power and authority to install peer-to-peer recognition programs. This will foster a sense of support and will promote healthy friendships as well.

You can also introduce innovative elements in those recognition programs, such as recognition cards. Nurses can write not only notes of appreciation but also feedback for their colleagues. It will foster a positive workplace decorated with lights of personalized notes of gratitude.

Celebratory Ceremonies and Occasions:

Being a nurse leader also means that you will have to organize celebratory occasions and ceremonies (no matter how small or large) to show your appreciation and recognition for your staff.

These ceremonies or events can take place outside the work setting as well. For example, you can arrange recognition breakfasts, annual reward events, annual dinners, or themed appreciation days or weeks. When you choose a themed appreciation week, you can add decorations as well. This chain of efforts will have a huge impact.

It will make these events memorable for the nurses and they will work passionately as a reward for your efforts. Also, a festive occasion is sometimes all a tired and exhausted mind needs to get refreshed and focused.

Underlining Personal and Professional Accomplishments:

When you are celebrating personal accomplishments, you are fostering a productive work environment. On the other hand, if you acknowledge the personal achievements of your staff, you build a meaningful network and healthy relationships.

Be it celebrating birthdays, annual work anniversaries, or academic goals, celebrating your staff's special days reflects that you are acknowledging the presence of your nurses more than individual beings.

Making a Wall of Appreciation:

In the prominent region of your workplace, you can fashion a "Wall of Appreciation". This wall will allow the colleagues to acknowledge and celebrate each other's win and victory together. You can suggest adding notes of appreciation, pictures, and achievements that will create a visual representation and add to the facility unit's aesthetics, too.

You need to update the wall of appreciation after regular periods of time to keep it evolving, fresh, and a permanent part of your leadership era.

Digital Appreciation Initiatives:

It is the age of technology, and you can benefit from advanced technology more than your profession requires. How can you use the digital world when it is not related to your work?

Besides using online platforms to establish networking, you can organize appreciative ceremonies online, too.

At many digital platforms like Zoom or Microsoft, you can hold these ceremonies where the members can send in their virtual expressions of appreciation and gratitude. The technology will help you inculcate various innovative elements in these ceremonies, such as you can make customized e-cards, virtual stickers, an audio full of appreciation, or even a video reflecting expressions of gratitude and appreciation.

These immediate and visual expressions of appreciation will help you foster the impacts of appreciation and build a good rapport with your organization.

Storytelling Sessions:

While organizing digital ceremonies or on-site events, you can include another innovative element in the form of the art of storytelling. You will offer an opportunity to your team members to share their unique success stories and experiences. You can also narrate their stories as a part of honoring their efforts.

The art of storytelling will not only be a testament of acknowledgment for their hard work but it will also inspire and motivate others. You will be able to harmonize deep and meaningful connections that surpass the formal or robotic interactions between all the workplaces.

It is obvious that these holistic approaches of appreciation and recognition rituals become successful through the art of communication. When you organize these ceremonies, you may notice that not everyone is good at or has mastered the art of effective communication.

Here, your role as a mentor comes in handy.

As a leader, you can guide them on how to express gratitude and share words of appreciation. You can provide your guidance in either short meetings or by handing over some useful written instructions.

This set of instructions must include the impact of active listening, showing genuine engagement, and gifting words of positive criticism.

This strategic approach will help you cultivate a positive work setting where appreciation is fostered regularly and authentically.

Implementation into Performance Evaluations:

While celebrating your team members' achievements, you also can make those achievements a part of your formal annual or monthly performance evaluations. Your evaluations will tell your team members that you value everyone's contribution to the landscape of the healthcare community.

This strategic inculcation will also help all the team members to understand that appreciation is neither an isolated nor occasional practice. Instead, it is woven into the fabric of the whole organization and feedback assessments.

Anonymous Recognition Options:

Some people prefer to offer their honest reviews when you inculcate the option of anonymous feedback.

The same goes for the recognition options. Some people prefer to embrace appreciation in some private form. It does not mean that you cannot hold those ceremonies for them. It simply means that you can acknowledge their appreciation on an individual level.

You can integrate anonymous recognition by using suggestion boxes or online platforms where nurses can express their gratitude without divulging their names.

Through self-reflection and problem-solving skills, this one act has comforted different personality types and ensured that everyone gets the chance to participate in a workplace where they will be appreciated.

In a nutshell, In the world of nursing leadership, dedication, commitment, and compassion lie at the heart of daily activities, and establishing a ritual of appreciation becomes more than a management strategy. In fact, It is one of the basic aspects of compassionate healthcare delivery. Through the acknowledgment, you will be able to enjoy many benefits in the form of continuous success in your leadership journey. Appreciation will boost the morale of your nursing team. They will not prefer to leave an environment where they feel appreciated and acknowledged. Ultimately, it will result in effective healthcare delivery and enhanced patient satisfaction.

Promoting Inclusivity and Diversity

When you foster a culture of positivity, you must acknowledge each person's presence regardless of their background. Therefore, it becomes vital to foster a diverse and inclusive culture. You can show affection and acknowledgment by establishing policies that cater to and support diversity and inclusivity by discouraging discrimination on the basis of sex, race, and ethnicity. It also fashions a sense of belonging and equality among all the employees.

Let us first explore the significance of inclusivity and diversity in a workplace:

Focusing on Patient Diversity:

Your team consists of individuals who have come from diverse backgrounds, each possessing distinctive linguistic, cultural, religious, and social traits. This diversity should only add to the efficiency of your team's success. If the team member is performing well, you should acknowledge their achievements despite their background or race.

In the healthcare facility, patients also come from diverse backgrounds. Inclusivity as well as diversity in the nursing workforce, can help you enhance the patient care and patient satisfaction rate. You can gently ask your team members who belong to the same background to take care of them. Simply, it will enhance patient satisfaction rates.

As a diverse workplace brings all the people together who have varied perspectives, expertise, and experiences, it also welcomes innovation, creativity, and efficiency. Moreover, having nurses from different backgrounds means that you can gain unique insights that can enhance the quality of patient-centered care.

In a workplace, Inclusivity refers to offering equal opportunities to all individuals. It also fosters a collaborative environment where every team member's strengths and power are recognized and perfectly utilized.

Reducing Health Disparities:

In the field of nursing, inclusivity and diversity lead to reducing health discrepancies. An inclusive nurse workforce becomes more responsive to the requirements of diverse patient populations and opens the doors for the development of intervention and institutional policies.

This proactive approach also assists in bridging the gaps between healthcare access and consequences.

Creating a Positive Work Setting:

When you foster a diverse and inclusive work environment, it brings positivity automatically. By forming a diverse and inclusive workplace, you make sure that your team feels heard, valued, and respected. It gifts them job satisfaction and helps them in their well-being.

Maintaining diversity and inclusivity can be challenging, but following these strategies can overcome this hurdle.

Cultural Competency Training:

As a nurse leader, you can offer cultural training to your staff and attend these cultural training sessions that will help you understand the importance of cultural diversity.

You can learn to navigate cultural challenges, build respect for other cultures, and learn to direct this cultural diversity in patient care through these training sessions.

Manifold Recruitment and Retention Techniques:

Have you thought about the fact that if you have diversity within your team, you will help your organization's reputation grow too?

As diverse people join your team, they will feel respected and valued. It will enhance the retention rate because no one wants to leave a place where their efforts lead to their professional success. Likewise, it will enhance your institution's reputation.

Employee Resource Groups (ERGs):

You can create Employee Resource Groups that can prove to be of a lot of help.

For instance, you have established an ERG for LGBTQ+ nurses. This supportive community offers networking opportunities and advocates for the rights of these people.

Employee Resource Groups also ensure that everyone may embrace a sense of belonging, help in fostering a supportive environment where they can share their experiences openly, and hence take the initiative to promote diversity.

Celebrating Cultural Competence:

You can also organize a cultural festival as a nurse leader who values diversity and inclusivity within your team.

When you organize annual cultural events, you need to allow different cultures and traditions to showcase their customs and narrate their stories of success. This will be entertaining and refreshing for all the people working in the healthcare community. Also, you will contribute to promoting a sense of unity.

This sense of unity will also be created when all of the workers, despite their backgrounds, work on one particular goal and go through the same working experiences.

In simple words, the celebrations underscore the significance of diversity and inclusivity as fundamental elements of the organization's culture.

Flexible Work Arrangements:

As a nurse leader, you can arrange a flexible schedule for your staff, but sometimes, it is not enough. However, introducing the option of flexible work arrangements can be useful.

You can ask and inform your organization to inculcate the option of flexible work arrangements. These arrangements can be in the form of remote work, hybrid options, or shortened work weeks. It can result in balancing work-life and enhancing the well-being of the community.

When necessary, your staff can avail the remote work option. Technology can help you stay in connection with your staff and their performance as well.

Time for Taking an Assessment :

- ↔ Before maintaining a culture of well-being, engage yourself in an assessment to evaluate your own physical and mental health and well-being.

- ↔ You need paper and a pen for this assessment.

- ↔ First of all, divide a page into two parts.

- ↔ The title of one side of the page would be Yes, and the other would be No.

- ↔ Now, ask yourself some questions related to your health. For instance, you can ask questions like:

- ↔ Do you take regular breaks?

- ↔ Can you keep your mind off work in your after-work routine?

- ↔ Do you let yourself be consumed by the workload?

- ↔ Can you maintain a balance between compassion and professionalism?

- ↔ If the answer is yes, write it on the yes side of the page. However, if the answer is no, write it in the other one.

- ↔ Moving to the next step, you will write all the possible solutions to all the Noes on the next page.

- ↔ Next time, when you work beyond your body's capacity, you will remember your mantra, which will help you take care of yourself.

In the last chapter, we will reflect on this transformative journey of nursing leadership and will highlight the most important aspects necessary for your continuous growth and impact in the leadership career.

Chapter 8

The Holistic Journey of Nursing Leadership

Your nursing leadership journey has nothing less than an evolving and transformative odyssey. As we have reached the destination of the leadership journey through this comprehensive guide, let us have a look at all the holistic approaches of this journey that form a long-lasting impact on your career, team, and the broader community of your healthcare.

In the ever-evolving landscape of nursing, for professionals, especially nurse leaders, continuous learning is a huge blessing in succeeding in their careers. Nursing leaders play a critical role in establishing the future of the healthcare industry. Their dedication to continuous professional advancement is mandatory for staying ahead of the healthcare organization. It also involves cultivating innovation and adapting to the changing needs of the healthcare system as well as of the nursing staff with resilience.

Let us explore the significance of embracing lifelong learning by getting insights into the arteries of continuous professional advancement through the power of a curious mind and the lens of adaptability.

Embracing Lifelong Learning:

Let us look at some of the benefits of embracing lifelong learning through this example.

The nursing leader, Rose O. Sherman, narrates a story about the time when she was teaching a leadership course named Nuts and Bolts Leadership in a large medical institution. At the same institution, she worked as the Head of Employee Education. She had the course designed for the new leaders but from all the disciplines of the hospital. During her teaching period, she got a call from one of the most senior leaders of the healthcare organization, and he asked for permission to take that course. Sherman informed him that the course is for beginning leaders, so he might have known all the strategies and content. However, if he wants to come, he is more than welcome.

With dedication and commitment to lifelong learning, he came to attend all five sessions (that consisted of 40 hours) of the course. When the course ended, he told her that he had learned a lot through this course and it would help him to become a great leader as well. He also showed his willingness to keep on learning throughout his leadership journey.

His deep words made me realize that leadership is not a destination; instead, it is a journey. Moreover, there is something to be learned again and again (Sherman, 2017).

After learning from this experience, let us explore some of the best ways and the significance of continuous learning in the field of nursing leadership.

Adapting to Technological Advancements:

Nursing leaders must stay updated regarding the changes in technological advancements in their healthcare industry as the healthcare landscape is prone to technological advancements, such as changes in electronic health records and telemedicine.

You can stay updated about these changes by continuing to learn about them through books or online platforms such as LinkedIn.

By staying informed about these changes, you can implement them in these healthcare facilities. Life-long learning about technological changes gives you an opportunity to enhance patient care delivery and facilitate operations.

Navigating Growing Healthcare Policies:

Like technologies, healthcare policies also undergo contact and regular waves of change. Therefore, it impacts the way patient care is managed.

As a nurse leader, you need to stay up to date about these changes so that you may ensure compliance and navigate through these challenges effectively.

It is through the art of continuous learning that grants you the skills and knowledge required to overcome these challenges.

Encouraging Evidence-Based Practice:

In the healthcare industry, nothing is more important than evidence-based practices. These evidence-based practices can be found in regularly published research papers.

As a nurse leader, you can not only read these papers to know about the latest trends in the industry but also contribute to these research papers. You can do so either through the power of knowledge, by conducting surveys, or by participating in the research.

Hence, lifelong learning helps you stay updated on the most recent scientific research.

Addressing Healthcare Disparities:

In your personal life, what do you do when you have to assemble a piece of furniture? You either seek help from the professionals or read the manual book.

Likewise, in the field of nursing, you can address most of the healthcare disparities through lifelong learning and education.

You can choose to learn about the social determinants of health, cultural aspects, and tools necessary to promote good quality health. You can read about these changes in scholarly articles and by attending seminars. Through this constant learning habit, you will be able to form new insights and implement healthcare policies more effectively that will entertain the needs of the diverse population of patients and nurse workforce.

Nurturing Leadership Skills:

Just like technological advances, leadership skills need continuous refinement. Through constant learning, you will be able to enhance your leadership skills, including but not limited to communication, problem-solving, and emotional intelligence.

The constant progression in such a role will contribute to effective team management and cultivating a positive work environment.

Avenues for Ongoing Professional Development in Nursing Leadership:

To continue your path toward professional development, you can use some of the continuous learning resources from these avenues:

Standard Education Programs:

Education is one of the powerful steps leading you to the land of successful leadership.

You can pursue any advanced medical degree or certificate according to your interest, or you can continue to work and pursue your education at the same time.

Professional Conferences and Seminars:

You can attend conferences and seminars that will help you stay informed and up to date regarding the latest trends in the healthcare industry.

These events will also provide you with opportunities for network building and gaining useful knowledge.

Online Learning Platforms:

The vast realm of the online world also entails many options for nursing leaders to grow and succeed. Among many other platforms, you can choose different topics and attain certificates via Linkedin Learning or Coursera.

These platforms and many others will help you shape your leadership journey based on your own and your career's needs, requirements, and interests.

Leadership Evolution Programs:

Several healthcare organizations provide tailored leadership development programs according to the needs of the nursing leaders.

These programs can be introduced via workshops, mentoring initiatives, and leadership coaching.

You can attend and engage in these programs to equip yourself with the guidance and knowledge of the senior leaders. You will also learn some strategies necessary to polish your leadership skills and overcome complex healthcare environments.

Cooperative Learning and Networking:

When it comes to learning new topics, your mentors and peers can help you in the process. You can join communications that appreciate collective learning. You can also join reading groups in your healthcare organization or online.

When you have learned these new skills, you always need to introduce these skills to your team members either through meetings or training sessions.

Cultivating a Mindset of Curiosity and Adaptability:

As you are going to contribute to cultivating a positive work ecosystem in the healthcare community, it is essential to inspire people to continue learning. As a nurse leader, you can foster an environment of continuous learning by promoting a mind of curiosity and adaptability.

Within your team, you can promote a mentality of adaptability and curiosity by encouraging risk-taking, developing effective communication, fostering a safe and healthy work environment, and creating opportunities.

Let us try to understand the importance of risk-taking as we have discussed all other factors in detail.

Within a professional setting, the quality of risk-taking emerges when there is no sense of fear or failure among your team members.

"The biggest risk is not taking any risk... In a world thats changing really quickly, the only strategy that is guaranteed to fail is not taking risks (Zuckerberg)."

Therefore, in the changing land of nursing, it is important for nurse leaders to take risks and encourage their teams to do so as well. Both of you can also help your whole organization grow, make all of the processes smooth, and ensure that you embrace success in your careers (Half, 2023).

As a nurse leader, you can build this risk-taking mindset in a lot of ways. First, you can introduce a culture of reward to empower your staff so that they may start integrating innovation into their tasks. When your team members take risks, you can reward them. This will also encourage others to contribute to the success of the whole organization. Second, you need to foster a positive culture that enhances job satisfaction. When there is job satisfaction, your team members will be open to taking calculated risks. Third, you can encourage your risk-taking members publicly, as it will motivate others to take risks. You can also organize weekly meetings where you can ask your team members to take risks by introducing new ideas. When they do so, you can appreciate them. This small step will inspire others to take risks. You can also suggest that they dedicate some of their time to brainstorming before working on a new learning project. Fourth, you will note that some of your team members are good at taking risks than others. Not only can you reward their innovative and curious minds, but you can also ask them to become mentors of innovation and adaptivity for others. Last, lead by example.

Whenever you introduce these risk-taking strategies to your team, make sure that you guide them through the S-M-A-R-T (Specific, measurable, achievable, relevant, and time-bound) approach.

Encourage a Learning Culture:

You can cultivate a learning culture through effective communication. For instance, you can highlight the impact of learning in their professional lives. You can tell them that they can learn more about the techniques of telemedicine or how to operate machinery easily by reading about it.

You can also suggest that they explore new perspectives that can add to the collective learning experience.

Set Personal Learning Goals:

Again, lead by example. You can align your personal objectives and relevant objectives with your professional ones. These goals can include learning about some skill or deepening your knowledge in a specific area of nursing.

You can revise these goals to ensure continuous growth.

You can also guide your team to do the same through your actions and experiences.

Value Feedback and Practice Self-Reflection:

You can look at the feedback to find areas of improvement. Likewise, you need to provide useful and constructive feedback to your team members. This feedback will provide opportunities to learn and grow.

You can also inculcate the activity of self-reflection.

Adopt Change and Innovation:

One of the main goals of acquiring long-term education is to embrace change and be open to innovation. As a nurse leader, you should focus on identifying those opportunities that help you implement new and innovative solutions to the challenges in the healthcare industry.

When you adopt these changes with the scalpel of knowledge and wear the uniform of adaptability, you not only empower others to face these challenges more easily but also contribute to a productive environment.

Participate in Communities of Practice:

You can also join communities of practice where you can rehearse your leadership skills by engaging in discussions. You can learn from the experiences of other professionals.

You need to encourage your team to engage in such communities, too.

We know that it seems like lifelong learning is a professional obligation. However, it is more than that. It is a certificate that leads you toward effective nursing leadership. It is a requirement for the landscape of nursing that keeps on growing and expanding day by day, and continuous learning is a way to make sure that you are prepared to face all of these changes. Similarly, formal education, such as pursuing an advanced degree in nursing or attaining a certificate, becomes tangible and interesting when you learn about these things by wearing the glasses of curiosity. In conclusion, lifelong learning is one of the powerful catalysts that lead to innovation, promise excellence, and deliver the best patient-centered care in the developing world of nursing leadership.

Balancing Compassion and Accountability:

Nursing leadership is a fragile balance between compassion and accountability. As a nurse leader, you will not only be responsible for delivering quality patient-centered healthcare but also for inspiring and empowering your team members.

Let us delve further into this delicate balance of compassion and accountability and how it helps in fostering a harmonious and effective leadership style.

In nursing, the essence of the compassionate leadership journey lies in empathy and understanding your patients, cultivating a healthy workplace, recognizing and valuing the efforts of your team members, and providing them with emotional help through effective communication.

Empathy and Understanding:

Compassionate leadership begins with empathy and understanding.

As a leader, you will come across many challenges where your team will feel low; you need to understand and show empathy.

You will communicate with them that you understand these challenges and will guide them along the way.

You can also show them your emotional support.

You can cultivate a positive environment by inspiring others to learn continuously, sharing and giving feedback, celebrating accomplishments, and addressing your teammates' concerns.

Through diversity and inclusion, each individual in your team will understand the importance of feeling helpful and valued. They will show respect as they receive it, so it will help you cultivate a positive environment.

The Need for Accountability in Nursing Leadership:

In simple words, accountability refers to the act of being responsible. In every career especially in the nursing career, the need for accountability is of immense significance.

There are certain factors that give rise to this need for accountability in the nursing leadership journey.

Patient Safety and Quality Care:

Accountability in the nursing profession is of prime importance as it ensures patient safety and delivers high-quality, patient-centered care.

As a nurse leader, you need to establish and implement these standards of practice to ensure that nursing care entails evidence-based guidelines and moral principles.

For nurse leaders, accountability becomes non-negotiable in maintaining the integrity of the quality delivery.

Professional Standards and Ethics:

As you know, great leaders lead by example, you, as a nurse leader, will be a demonstration upholding professional ideals and ethical principles in their teams.

Accountability encompasses the implementation of adherence to the principles of morals, ethics, and compliance and addressing everything that deviates from set norms and standards.

This commitment to the ethical code of conduct adds to the trustworthiness of the field of nursing.

Legal and Regulatory Compliance:

As a nurse leader, you will ensure that your team will adhere to all the legal and regulatory requirements. This way you will be able to keep your team on the right course so that they may work more vigilantly.

Adherence to the legal requirements involves staying informed about the recent variations in law and regulations, organizing training programs necessary for education, and addressing any confusion or compliance issues immediately.

You can also communicate with your team members about the consequences of failure to meet these legal requirements. You can tell them that failure to meet these standards can result in severe penalties for both the individuals and the healthcare community.

The Need for Accountability in Nursing Leadership:

Resource Management and Efficiency:

In your nursing leadership career, you will have to manage resources, including but not limited to staffing, equipment, and budgeting. While dealing with resource management, your responsibility is to make strategic decisions that will enhance both the efficiency and quality of patient care.

Managing resources and their efficiency can be very challenging, and therefore, you need to be very open about the resource constraints with your staff so that you may all work together to deal with these challenges effectively.

Performance and Continuous Improvement:

The continuous improvement stems from continuous work opportunities and feedback. As a nurse leader, you know that accountability in your profession involves assessing individual as well as team performance.

Besides cultivating clear and transparent expectations, you need to offer constructive feedback. You can address all the performance issues and their resolutions in your feedback.

You can also build a culture of constant improvement by identifying the regions of growth, implementing useful strategies, and evaluating the consequences of these changes. After evaluating the outcomes of these strategies, you can implement those changes that enhance the overall efficiency of nursing practice.

135

Legal and Regulatory Compliance:

As a nurse leader, you will also be responsible for ensuring that your team complies with legal requirements.

You need to make sure that you invest in training and meetings to comply with the legal and regulatory requirements if the policies change.

Harmonizing Compassion and Accountability in Nursing Leadership

Let us now learn to harmonize both compassion and accountability into our nursing leadership.

Establishing Clear Expectations:

The key to maintaining and balancing compassion and accountability starts by setting clear expectations. You need to communicate expectations regarding performance, behavior, adherence to legal requirements, and professional principles clearly. You also need to make sure that they understand their responsibilities and do not undermine the significance of accountability while fulfilling their duties.

For example, you have come to know about a new policy that requires adherence to protocols regarding infection control. As a nurse leader, what aspects would you communicate with your team members regarding this change?

You need to guide them to ensure the critical nature of patient safety. You also need to inform them about the role expected from them in maintaining a sterile and safe work environment.

Cultivating a Learning Culture:

As a compassionate leader, you will have to create a learning culture where your fellow nurses will feel comfortable when acknowledging their errors and mistakes so that they may learn from their mistakes. This compassionate approach will also foster a sense of accountability in your team.

Let us understand this through one example. Being a nurse leader, you have noticed a medication administration error. To deal with this situation, you can conduct a meeting with the concerned nurse and understand the contributing factors that led to the errors. Compassionately, you will also guide your nurse to report such incidents immediately and will offer her additional training or instructions regarding medication safety. This meeting will help you establish a sense of accountability within your team.

Providing Constructive Feedback:

Again, positive, constructive feedback can also help in a workplace setting. You need to highlight shortcomings and skills that are required for improved performance rather than blaming the concerned person. If you see that the members need more training, provide them with additional training sessions.

Promoting a Just Culture:

What is a just culture? A just culture believes that errors or mistakes are the results of system failures instead of individual negligence.

As a nurse leader, you need to establish and maintain a just and fair system. You can do so by addressing these systematic errors while holding the concerned individuals accountable for their actions at the same time. Thai proactive approach will help you maintain the required balance between accountability and compassion by maintaining patient safety.

When any mishap or incident may happen, as a leader of the nurses, you should promptly run an analysis of the root cause of an incident. This way you will be able to identify the root cause of system issues. At the same time, you will collaborate with your staff to implement changes as well. Through this collaboration, you will be able to view this incident as an opportunity to grow.

It is an ongoing and continuous process to maintain the balance between compassion and accountability in nursing leadership. Compassionate leaders always acknowledge and value the humanity of their team members, provide them emotional support when they need it, cultivate healthy, supportive work environments, and promote individual well-being. Simultaneously, they ensure adherence to law requirements, working standards, and the delivery of safe and quality patient-centered care through accountability.

Legacy Building in Nursing Leadership:

The idea of legacy in the dynamic field of nursing goes beyond the achievements of titles in your professional life. It entails all the changes that have been implemented positively, all the lives that have been professionally informed, and the positive culture that has become a part of the nursing community.

But this makes us wonder what legacy is.

A nursing legacy is about producing, maintaining, and inspiring a culture of excellence and well-being. It translates to taking an oath to achieve the highest standards of patient care and keep on learning throughout the journey.

By setting and leading the examples of excellence, you, as a nurse leader, will be able to influence your team and organization, inviting people to seek inspiration from your legacy of quality, innovation, and success.

It is up to you to leave any type of legacy behind you. For instance, you can leave behind a legacy of valuing and supporting a positive culture based on excellence. This should include commitment and dedication to the highest patient standards, continuous learning, and helping each other. When you set the expectations of excellence and success, you will inform the behaviors and the mindset of your entire team, leaving behind a legacy of quality, unity, collaboration, and innovation.

One of the most important nursing leader's legacy is the progression of patient care. You can prioritize the well-being and delivery of patient care. By achieving your legacy, you will be able to contribute to a healthy work environment where empathy and compassion go hand in hand with patient care. This patient-care legacy mirrors not only a strong commitment to enhancing the patient satisfaction rate but also to holistic well-being.

Similarly, a long-lasting legacy in the field of nursing leadership entails a passion for mentorship and the art of guiding future nurses. You can invest in the growth of your team members by offering them training or necessary assistance. By mentorship, you are ensuring that your influence surpasses the realm of your own professional life and enters into other lives and the fabric of your organization.

The upcoming leaders will also pass on your legacy by providing the necessary guidance, training, and assistance to those in need.

As a nurse leader, you will wear the mask of resilience and wear the uniform of adaptability from time to time. Your adaptability and resilience will show nothing but your commitment to cultivating positive organizational change. This is the legacy of forward-thinking, and it is one of the first legacies that become proactive strategies for your upcoming generations of nurses.

In a nutshell, all these forms of legacies will help you extend your influence beyond yourself.

Now, let us have a glimpse of some of the positive changes that you might have implemented:

As a nurse leader, you conducted training sessions and meetings on evidence-based practices so that you might empower your team to value their profession and also encourage them to critically assess new research findings. After evaluating the new findings, you guided them to instill those new protocols into their daily routines.

As a nurse leader, you have also embraced the transformative journey by constantly staying up to date with all new technological changes.

You have built professional networking that helps you advance toward your career goals.

Time For The Activity:

- ↔ Create a vision board and name it Legacy Vision Board.

- ↔ It should encapsulate your aspirations and goals.

- ↔ You can add the list of legacies that you want to leave behind.

- ↔ Decorate it with visuals and pictures.

This visual representation of your Legacy Vision Board will be your reminder of the legacy of your nursing leadership.

Conclusion

The Journey to Nursing Leadership starts with finding the potential of leadership hidden in yourself and continuing to use and enhance those skills so that you may continue to advance in your career. Once you have reached your career goals, you will know that it is not the end of your success; rather, it is the beginning of many successes.

From identifying your leadership style to embracing your leadership style, from adopting your leadership skills (effective communication, adaptability, and resilience) to adopting proactive leadership strategies (building a positive environment), and from knowing the impact of empathy to accountability, we have learned the essence of nursing leadership.

Through *Empower Your Nursing Leadership*, you have come to know that the pearls of wisdom ingrained in leadership skills will not only make you a good leader but also show its impact on your surrounding sphere of healthcare. You know that as a nurse leader or nurse manager, you have the potential to contribute to the whole healthcare organization. This legacy of contribution, along with your impactful leadership, will keep on inspiring and empowering many upcoming generations of nursing. Moreover, you will become a part of a transformative movement where your compassion and empowered leadership skills will lead to a positive landscape of change, a land where nursing will be synonymous with excellence, growth, and empathy.

It is through your skills that you cultivate a positive work environment that leads to success. Always remember that a positive workplace is one where efforts are appreciated, all kinds of concerns are addressed, and empathy and accountability echo. It is also the power of your clear and effective communication skills that leads to a collaborative and supportive environment.

When you are embarking on the journey of successful leadership, you should always keep the toolkit of continuous learning with yourself. You can learn either by pursuing an advanced degree or certificate or by attending some training programs or workshops. It is through continuous learning that you open the doors to new opportunities, and it also helps you tackle some of the challenges and obstacles as well.

In the search for leadership excellence, the purpose of pursuing education is more than acquiring knowledge. It is about embodying those learnings into your actions. Throughout this journey, you have expressed the willingness to understand the purpose of education and continuous learning and to implement them into your professional life. Your dedication and enthusiasm are also a testament to your leadership standards.

As a nurse leader, you will also create an environment where continuous education and learning are appreciated. This proactive approach will help your team understand the impact of constant learning and staying updated regarding the latest trends in the healthcare industry.

When you inject your positive leadership skills to create a positive and collaborative environment, you also contribute to the entire organization, and your legacy of leadership sleeps on evolving and motivating others.

So, if you want to achieve success in your leadership or you want to become an aspiring nursing leader, start your journey now. You can not only understand the obstacles that will hinder your path toward success but also be able to overcome these challenges by implementing the strategies mentioned in the book.

The book Empower Your Nursing Leadership is a roadmap that is tailored to meet the challenging and evolving needs of the dynamic world of nursing and the healthcare system in general. Be it any phase in your nursing leadership journey; you can pass that phase successfully through this book. You will feel relatable to this book not only because it talks about all the challenges, including but not limited to communication, inclusivity, and managing diverse perspectives, but also because the author of the book, Brandy Covington, has penned down her own experiences and approaches that guarantee success. It is a gift for woman, by a woman, who believes that leadership is found in everyone equally. Fun fact: 90% of nurses are female, with a staggering male population rising in the field.

Without any further delay, align your short-term and long-term goals and design your roadmap towards success. If you need any help along the way, you can apply and implement the strategies present in the book.

When you start to thrive in your nursing profession, you need to empower others as well. As a nurse leader, your success will depend on the success of your team, and therefore, you need to be a compassionate, considerate, and transformational leader.

As we conclude this comprehensive guide to nursing leadership, remember that your journey to nursing leadership is ongoing and continuous. It will not end unless you achieve your goal. Afterward, a new journey of success will be waiting for you.

In your journey, know that through the potential of continuous learning, building a positive environment, maintaining the balance between accountability and compassion, and building strong networks, you are more than a nurse leader; you are a catalyst that brings positivity and innovation in the realm of healthcare.

Thank you so much for being a part of this empowering journey. I want to express my gratitude for your steady commitment to personal and professional advancement. Your dedication to refining your skills and expertise, shows its the very step in your leadership journey, and it also shows that you are ready to be a transformational leader.

Throughout this guidebook, we have uncovered the nuances of successful leadership and delved deeper into the practices and strategies that demonstrate inspirational leaders. Your involvement merged with your passion for learning has been palpable, and it is this very commitment that fueled this essence of leadership exploration.

As we end this book of our mutual leadership journey, you are invited to stay connected. Just like the dynamic and evolving world of leadership, our dedication to growth and development must be equally dynamic. By choosing to stay together, you allow us to keep you updated with all the upcoming resources, latest trends, and deep insights so that you may enrich your nursing leadership journey.

Lastly, I extend my deepest gratitude for letting me be a stimulus or a part of your leadership journey. May your journey to effective leadership be pregnant with continuous developments, deep and healthy connections, and unmatched success.

References

Ali, M. (2013). *Soul of a butterfly: reflections on life's journey.* Simon & Schuster

Contributor, N. T. (2017, February 15). *"As a nurse leader, your role is to empower your team."* Nursing Times. https://www.nursingtimes.net/archive/as-a-nurse-leader-your-role-is-to-empower-your-team

HALF, R. (2023, August 29). *9 ways to encourage a workplace culture of calculated risks.* ROBERT HALF. https://www.roberthalf.com/au/en/insights/management-tips/9-ways-encourage-workplace-culture-calculated-risks

hannahnightingale2020. (2019, August 29). *Stories of nurse leaders.* Nursing Now. https://archive.nursingnow.org/bongi-sibanda-i-am-truly-grateful-for-this-challenge-that-keeps-me-curious-and-looking-for-ways-to-serve-better-daily/

Helio Fred Garcia. (2012). *The power of communication*Irresistible: *skills to build trust, inspire loyalty, and lead effectively.* Ft Press.

Maraboli, S. (2014). *Life, the truth, & being free.* A Better Today.

Nucleus_AI. (2023, May 24). *THE BIGGEST RISK IS NOT TAKING ANY RISK.* Your story._HYPERLINK "https://yourstory.com/2023/05/embracing-risk-zuckerbergs-philosophy" HYPERLINK "https://yourstory.com/2023/05/embracing-risk-zuckerbergs-philosophy" HYPERLINK "https://yourstory.com/2023/05/embracing-risk-zuckerbergs-philosophy"HYPERLINK "https://yourstory.com/2023/05/embracing-risk-zuckerbergs-philosophy" HYPERLINK "https://yourstory.com/2023/05/embracing-risk-zuckerbergs-philosophy" HYPERLINK "https://yourstory.com/2023/05/embracing-risk-zuckerbergs-philosophy" HYPERLINK "https://yourstory.com/2023/05/embracing-risk-zuckerbergs-philosophy" HYPERLINK "https://yourstory.com/2023/05/embracing-risk-zuckerbergs-philosophy"https://yourstory.com/2023/05/embracing-risk-zuckerbergs

Orlin, B. (2019). *Change Is the Only Constant.* Hachette UK.

O. Sherman, R. (2017, August 17). *Leaders Should be Lifelong Learners.* Emerging RN Leader. https://emergingrnleader.com/leaders-lifelong-learners/

Sadler, F. (2023, May 19). *7 Leadership Styles in Nursing — Which Is Yours?* Relias. https://www.relias.com/blog/7-leadership-styles-in-nursing

Tracy, B. (2012). *The Power of Self-Confidence: Become Unstoppable, Irresistible, and Unafraid in Every Area of Your Life.* John Wiley & Sons, Inc.

Wood, R. (2021). *Transforming Leadership.* Nih.gov; National Academies Press (US). https://www.ncbi.nlm.nih.gov/books/NBK209867/

Additional Resources

Besides Empower Your Nursing Leadership, you can refine your journey to nursing leadership by reading the following book or article or attending conferences. All these resources will help you advance toward your career goal and professional achievements.

Provide a list of recommended books, articles, online courses, or conferences related to nursing leadership and career advancement. Encourage readers to explore these resources for continued learning and professional development.

Book: "Dare to Lead" by Brené Brown - Link: *https://a.co/d/iWKuqAp*

Takeaway: In this book, you will learn about valiant leadership and the impact of vulnerability from distinguished researcher Brené Brown.

Article: "The Power of Reflective Leadership" - Link: *https://amara.fi/the-power-of-reflection-in-leadership/*

Takeaway: Delve deeper into the impacts and influence of reflective leadership on personal as well as professional growth.

Online Course: "Effective Networking for Healthcare Leaders" - Link: *https://www.udemy.com/share/101IFa/*

Takeaway: With the help of this online course, you can hone the networking skills designed for healthcare managers.

Conference: National Nursing Leadership Summit - Link: *https://brinetwork.com/2024-nursing-leadership-summit/*

Takeaway: You can join this annual conference to not only connect with your healthcare leaders but also gain knowledge about the industry's latest trends. You can also hone and polish your leadership skills.

Connect with the Author

After reading the book Empower Your Nursing Leadership by Brandy Covington, if you have any questions or feedback, or you want to share your leadership journey with her, you can contact her via email, LinkedIn, Twitter, and the Website.

Email: www.covington.brandy@icloud.com

LinkedIn: www.linkedin.com/in/brandysnotaryservice

Instagram: www.instagram.com/8randyCovington/

Facebook: www.facebook.com/8randycovington/

I also encourage you to be an active participant in your community: a community full of aspirational leaders committed to bringing positive change and empowering other leaders around them.

Let us learn, grow, evolve, and shape our future of leadership together.

Acknowledgments

As we embrace the culmination of this transformation journey, it is with immense humility that I express my gratitude and appreciation to all those people and organizations whose steady and constant support, along with their contributions, have helped me write this empowering book. Thank you for all of your help.

First of all, I would like to extend my heartful gratitude to my Lord Jesus Christ and to my guides and mentors; it is through their wisdom and guidance that I am able to shape my journey and experiences in an impactful manner. In fact, your dedication to cultivating growth has inspired and shaped my personal as well as professional advancement.

I would also like to express my thanks to my peers and fellows who have shared their expertise and perspectives throughout this journey. The supportive air that permeated our discussions and meetings has enriched the content and ensured that the subjects are addressed properly. Our collaborative commitment has been one of the driving forces behind the success and completion of this project.

I am thankful for all the professionals who took the time to help me get through when I had difficulties writing this book. Your willingness to share your deep insights has added to the authenticity and credibility of this project, for which I am deeply grateful.

To all my family and friends, who contributed to this empowering journey through their unparalleled and constant encouragement and understanding during this writing journey. Thank you so much for being the support that has sustained my spirit throughout and helped me achieve the goal of this book.

This book stands as a testimony to the collective and collaborative efforts of the leader community who strives for an excellent leadership career. This book has been woven into the fabric of healthcare essence and excellence.

Share Your Thoughts and Feelings About Your Experience

Hey there, amazing nurses!

Here's how you, yes YOU, can write a review on Amazon:

What's cool about the book: Think about the parts of the book that you really liked. Maybe it taught you something new or gave you awesome ideas. Share those cool things!

How does it help you be a leader: Did you try something from the book in real life, like at the hospital or clinic? Tell everyone how it went! Did it make you a better leader?

Keep it simple: Just like talking to a friend, you can keep your words simple and clear. Explain why you think other nurses should read this book too.

Remember, your words can help other nurses decide if they want to read the book. Your superpower of words can make a big difference! ✦

Cheers,

Brandy Covington